Mary Ann Cotton

ARTHUR APPLETON

Mary Ann Cotton

Her Story and Trial

First published in Great Britain by
Michael Joseph Ltd
1973
This edition specially produced by Cedric Chivers Ltd., Bristol
for the publisher **County Durham Books**
Durham County Council
Arts, Libraries & Museums Dept.
County Hall, Durham DH1 5TY

ISBN 1 897585 24 1

Printed in Great Britain by
Cromwell Press Ltd., Broughton Gifford, Wilts.
Bound by Cedric Chivers Ltd., Bristol

Mary Ann Cotton
She's dead and she's rotten
She lies in her bed
With her eyes wide oppen.
Sing, sing, oh, what can I sing
Mary Ann Cotton is tied up with string.
Where, where? Up in the air
Sellin' black puddens a penny a pair.

Children's Rhyme

The time you speak of my dark eyes i wos happy then, and them Wos days of joy to all of our soles . . .

From a Letter written by Mary Ann Cotton in Durham gaol

Contents

	Prologue	11
ONE	West Auckland	13
TWO	The first hearing: August, 1872	21
THREE	Three more at Bishop Auckland: February, 1873	31
FOUR	The story before West Auckland	47
FIVE	The Durham Spring Assizes: March, 1873	68
SIX	The numbered days	102
SEVEN	The hanging	118
EIGHT	A summing up	135
	Sources and Acknowledgements	147
	Index	151

List of Illustrations

The actuality . . . taken by a Durham city photographer when Mary Ann was in custody in 1872 or 1873 *facing page* 64

And the representation

In 1872 this was Townend's chemist's shop by West Auckland green 65
Darlington Road, West Auckland. The original name, Johnson Terrace, was on the square namestone near the roof
20, Johnson Terrace: Mary Ann Cotton's first home in West Auckland

The back of Johnson Terrace 96
Frontage of Durham goal and assize courts. (By kind permission of the *Sunderland Echo*)

The Governor of Durham gaol to the Home Secretary. (Transcript of Crown-copyright record H.O. 45/9314/14514/10 in the Public Record Office, which appears by permission of the Controller of H.M. Stationery Office). 97

Prologue

People just stared at her now. They were waiting outside the station and on the platform. They had murmured when her cab arrived and the three of them had got out; four, counting the precious baby, but now they just clustered near, silent.

She was notorious now . . . deep in winter: in the cold – although they gave her a good fire, in the place she had just left. The trees around here were black-brown, leafless, as they were in the valley of the Wear below: the grass was wet, sodden, browny.

Below there were the piled-up houses, sloping gardens, the grey castle on its hill; and the cathedral, its thick central tower stubbing upwards. All was set, firm, still, solid on the earth, without movement, as if it were impossible that life-ending movements could ever be twitched into action, could ever happen, could ever be allowed to happen, not only here, down below, but anywhere.

Her fingers caressed her precious baby, and the man and woman who flanked her tried to talk naturally. There was a movement and a comment at the back of the people . . . perhaps about the baby. A bit odd, perhaps they thought, that she appeared to love this baby, and had even lived longer because of it . . . No, God, no, they couldn't do it . . . they couldn't do that after she had been in their care so long, and had got to know them. They couldn't make her walk to it, in the cold early morning, chilly, damp, shivering . . . Lord, have mercy. They wouldn't do that while she had the baby. She must hold on to it.

They – the gazers – who had expected to gaze at a cruel appearance, saw a woman who looked as if she could be kindly. She was neat, clean, with fine dark eyes; above medium height – withdrawn, of course, now, withdrawn and subjugated in her special state. And how men had liked her! And she must have liked men. Four husbands, twelve children, forty years old, and yet, not so long ago – and she had little money – three men had been willing to marry her. One was the father of the baby. And one was dead, but he was the powerful one.

The 8.28 train came in. They found the right compartment. They put her between them. Comforting the child she gazed out at the countryside, the bare woods, streams, hills, and farms, and at the pits and pit villages and pit-heaps. Her escorts would exclaim at the sight of the people waiting to see her at every little station: sometimes they would lean forward so that the people couldn't see her easily, at other times they didn't bother. They talked gently, told of funny and odd happenings: she laughed two or three times.

Then, at last, there was the long slow turning into Bishop Auckland station. There were more people than ever, silent again, and policemen. Clutch the child. Along the platform, through the archway, and there at the entrance an omnibus was waiting. All the long way up Newgate Street, people stood waiting to see her, and along Bondgate too. Behind, and sometimes at the sides, boys danced and shouted.

She was not far now from quiet, pleasant West Auckland, with its long green restful views. The sound and sight of its cricket matches on the green. Lovely in deep summer . . . Dark, so dark at night. She had only two summers there . . . when she had been free.

CHAPTER ONE

West Auckland

You don't mean to tell me that this little healthy fellow is going to die?

Mary Ann Cotton came to West Auckland in the summer of 1871, with her husband, Frederick; their baby born in the January; and two children, both boys, of her husband's former marriage. Cotton had been a hewer at North Walbottle, a few miles west of Newcastle, and he continued at this work at West Auckland colliery. He was about the same age as Mary Ann and one can be next-to-certain he would not know he was her fourth husband. At their marriage in the old church of St Andrew's in Newcastle on 17th September, 1870, she gave the name of Mowbray, that of her deceased first husband and the only one with whom she lived for a long time. The marriage with Cotton was a bigamous one for her, as her third husband, James Robinson, a Sunderland shipwright, was still alive.

In West Auckland they lived in Johnson Terrace, now called Darlington Road, almost certainly at number twenty. Joseph Nattrass, an old friend and probably an old lover of Mary Ann's, was living in the same street. He was four years younger than Mary Ann, recently widowed, and he lodged with a family called Shaw. He was also a hewer at the West Auckland colliery. One can assume that, with Frederick Cotton unsuspecting, Joseph Nattrass living at West Auckland was the main reason for the move there.

On 19th September, 1871, some two months after coming to the village, Frederick Cotton, after suffering severe pains at work, died fairly suddenly. He was thirty-nine and had been married to Mary Ann for a year and two days. His doctor certified that he thought death was due to gastric fever.

A respectable-looking three months or so later Nattrass moved into Mary Ann's house as a lodger. Within a few weeks it was understood they were to marry: later it was stated that they 'cohabited'. But, direfully for Nattrass, Mary Ann had been a nurse and she was asked to look after a Mr Quick-Manning who had gone down with smallpox in his lodgings at Brookfield Cottage, a superior house in Johnson Terrace. He was excise officer at the large brewery in West Auckland, and higher up the social scale than Mary Ann and her pitmen. Pitmen were very nearly at the bottom. He was impressed by Mary Ann; the relationship became a loving one; the pair of them talked of marriage. There followed a clearance of human impedimenta.

In the space of three weeks, from 10th March to 1st April. Easter Monday, 1872, there were three more deaths in Mary Ann's home: Cotton's elder boy, also called Frederick, ten years old; Mary Ann's own child, the baby, Robert Robson Cotton, (named after her brother,) fourteen months; and Nattrass. Nattrass and young Frederick were said to have died of fever, and the baby of convulsions from teething.
Within a fortnight of Nattrass's death Mary Ann was pregnant by the excise officer.

She had taken two other lodgers, brothers called Taylor, but there were no emotional bonds with them. One of the Taylors was still with her when she and the remaining child moved to 13, Front Street early in May. This was, and is, a three-storeyed, stone-built house on the northern side of the green. There is a flag-stoned floor and only one room on each floor. The upper rooms were then reached by a ladder resting against the lip of an opening cut in the floor above. These openings could be covered by boarding. The second Taylor soon left her, and with the exception of another lodger, with her for only a week, she was alone with the child, seven-year-old Charles Edward.

Although Cotton and Nattrass had each left her all they had, their tough physical graft had not earned much, and she received only one and sixpence a week relief money for the boy. There was gossip now in the village that she and the excise officer would be marrying, but the weeks slipped by.

The assistant overseer in West Auckland was Thomas Riley who ran a corner general merchant shop on the other side of the green from Mary Ann. On Saturday, 6th July, he called on Mary Ann to see if she would look after another smallpox patient. She said she couldn't because of Charles Edward. She had written to the boy's uncle in Ipswich to see if he would take him, and she had offered to supply some clothing, but the uncle wouldn't take him. Although the little boy was there as she spoke she told Riley she was much tied by him, and then she asked if Riley would give her an order for the boy to be put into the workhouse. Riley said he could give her one for the boy only if she went in with him. Mary Ann said she would never go into such a place. It was hard on her, she said, to keep the boy when he was not her own, especially when she had an opportunity of taking in a respectable lodger. Riley laughed and asked if the lodger would be Quick-Manning. He had heard that he and she might marry, he said. Mary Ann smiled and said, 'It might be so. But the boy is in the way.' Then she added, 'Perhaps it won't matter, as I won't be troubled long. He'll go like all the rest of the Cotton family.'

Riley put out his hand to Charles Edward.

'You don't mean to tell me that this little healthy fellow is going to die?'

'He'll not get up,' she observed. Riley understood her to mean by this that the boy would not live to manhood.

Early the following Friday, 12th July, at about six in the morning, Riley, passing near Mary Ann's house, saw her standing just inside the doorway. She seemed to be distressed, and he went over to see her.

'My boy's dead,' she said.

'You don't mean to tell me that the little fellow I was talking to, that he's dead?'

She nodded. 'Will you come in and see him?'

Riley shook his head. He was shocked, suddenly hostile and highly suspicious, and, early as it was, he went straight to the village police office and saw Sergeant Tom Hutchinson. A little later he went to see Dr Kilburn. The doctor was surprised to hear of the boy's death. He had seen him twice the previous day, and Dr Chalmers, his assistant, had seen the boy three times during the week. Riley expressed his suspicion so forcibly that Kilburn decided he would postpone making out a death certificate.

Not obtaining a certificate that Friday was the first blow Mary Ann received. She had let the Prudential agent know of the death, but when he called with the £4 10s. 0d. insurance money, which she needed, he would not hand it over as she had no certificate.

Sergeant Hutchinson waited on Dr Kilburn and when the doctor confirmed that he was not prepared to certify the cause of death Hutchinson reported the case to the coroner. Kilburn requested permission to carry out a post-mortem, and the corner ordered an inquest to be held the next day, on the Saturday afternoon, 13th July.

On the Saturday morning Hutchinson told Mary Ann that an inquest was to be held.

'For why?'

'Dr Kilburn won't issue a burial certificate.'

'People are saying I poisoned the child,' she said, 'but I am in the clear.' They were saying that, she said, because they had heard she had tried to get the boy into the workhouse. Then she re-told her sorry tale – with no reported sorrow for the child – of writing to the boy's uncle, 'up south'; of being only his stepmother; of how he had prevented her from earning many a pound. 'I've had a great deal of trouble with the Cotton family,' she concluded, 'with so many of them dying in such a short time.'

There had been sympathy for Mary Ann when Frederick Cotton died so soon after coming to the village, leaving her with three children, two of them not her own. There were reports that there was a subscription for her, that the colliery owners, Pease and Partners, contributed, let her have free coal and allowed her to live rent free for a time. This sympathy began to drain away when it became obvious that Nattrass was taking Cotton's place, and then the time spent later with Quick-Manning caused further comment. Then there was the succession of deaths. Riley, who saw Mary Ann regularly about relief payments, was the first man of authority to be suspicious.

The inquest was held at the Rose and Crown public house, next door to Mary Ann's home in Front Street, before the deputy coroner, Thomas Dean. The decisive evidence was Kilburn's. But he, with Chalmers, began the post-mortem examination – on a table in Mary Ann's house – only an hour before the inquest and because of this he arrived uncertain. He had found nothing to indicate poisoning. He said death could have been from natural causes – he thought gastro-enteritis. When pressed by jurymen to give a definite opinion, he could not. The jury, after being out for an hour, returned a verdict of death by natural causes.

Mary Ann seemed to be cleared. Relieved, she spoke bitterly to Riley. Riley, however, was unrepentant. He refused to accept the verdict. He not only thought, but also continued to maintain that she had poisoned the boy. Later she wrote of him, '. . . as fore Riley god Will juge him, not A orthely Juge.'

She wrote to him now, after the inquest, saying that as overseer he could see to the boy's funeral expenses, as she couldn't.

Riley did this, and little Charles Edward was buried on the Monday at the expense of the parish.

But the holding of the inquest, in spite of the verdict, fanned talk about Mary Ann. On the Monday, the *Newcastle Journal*, reporting the inquest, exploded the information that there was talk in West Auckland that Mary Ann Cotton was a wholesale poisoner. The inquest, the paper said, had been held as a consequence of this talk and the apparently unnatural death of the boy. There were also rumours that Mary Ann had not been at home when the boy died, that she spent the night elsewhere.

There is no record that Mary Ann received support of any kind from Quick-Manning – their unborn child was to more than make up for this – although her preoccupation with the excise officer prior to the death of Charles Edward was made evident when a man called William Lowrey, a stranger in West Auckland, asked if he could lodge with her. She needed his board money, but she hesitated because of what Quick-Manning would say. She eventually agreed, only to tell Lowrey a day or two later that he would have to go as the gentleman she was going to marry did not like her taking in men lodgers. Lowrey was in the house a week. Mary Ann would already have told him she did not want him to stay when she made her unwise comments to Riley on the Saturday. On the Monday when Lowrey was leaving Mary Ann mentioned to him that her boy had turned poorly.

Lowrey said he never saw her behave unkindly to the boy. During the week he had listened sympathetically to her resentment at what the neighbours were saying. This means there was talk against her before the death of Charles Edward. There was suspicion in the gossip, which Riley, meeting people, would have heard. For Mary Ann to go ahead with a further death was a foolish and desperate and arrogant act.

Quick-Manning would be shocked and frightened at the eruption of feeling against Mary Ann on the death of Charles Edward. He would fear people thought he was implicated, and so he was, for he provided a motive for the child's death. He could well have laid down that he was not prepared to marry when it meant supporting a child of another man and woman. Who is to know how firm he was? And when, for Mary Ann, the boy stood in the way not only of marriage, but also of taking a nursing job, thoughts about poisoning could have started. There must have been restraint in Quick-Manning's feelings about Mary Ann, otherwise he would have gone into her house as a lodger even with the boy there. If she had done nothing, she might have got what she wanted in the end, when her obvious child-bearing condition put enough social pressure on Quick-Manning to cause him to marry her.

But after the inquest, in that miserable last week of freedom, Mary Ann would know that Quick-Manning was finished with her. There was no compassionate act by him. She had moved around the North East a lot and now, she decided, was the time to be moving again. But she had no money. Surely Quick-Manning would have let her have some so that she could get away. But perhaps the two could not face each other. She went to Lowrey and said he could have all her furniture for ten pounds. He advised her not to leave, saying that if she did it would make it look as if all the stories about her were true. He didn't convince her, but he spread doubt in her; his words carried away her urgency, fatally for her.

Lowrey bought some of the furniture and said he would sell the rest for her. Mary Ann went back home. Her head began to ache and a sore throat began and she took to the seeming refuge of her bed. This was on the Tuesday. One woman friend remained, old Mrs Dodds, who had lived next door in Johnson Terrace, and Mary Ann asked her to go for the doctor. Neither Kilburn nor Chalmers would come to see her and Chalmers said she should go elsewhere now for medical attention.

But Mary Ann could well have felt that this was merely a bad time, an uncomfortable time, to be got over. She had been cleared at the inquest; the boy was buried and, although there was gossip of other poisonings, because of that inquest verdict there was no real reason to do any digging up in St Helen's church graveyard. After a day or two she acted again about leaving when she gave her best clothing to Mrs Dodds to put in pawn for her: there were some silk dresses and a fine paisley shawl which had cost five pounds.

If Mary Ann had known of what was left in Dr Kilburn's house along the street she would have fled West Auckland, even without money. During his hasty post-mortem autopsy Kilburn had not given himself time to make any chemical examination, but so that he could do so later if he felt he should or was asked to do so, he put the stomach and other viscera in a closet which he locked. Neither coroner nor jury asked for a chemical analysis. On the Sunday he poured the contents of the stomach, five fluid ounces, into a jar which he retained; the rest was buried in the garden.

On the Wednesday the doctor submitted part of the stomach contents to a rough test for arsenic, known as Reinsch's test, a method first shown in 1842 by a German chemist, Hugo Reinsch. In this, suspected fluid is boiled with hydrochloric acid and a piece of clean copperfoil is added. If arsenic is there a deposit forms on the copper. Kilburn, to his horror, regret and dismay, I think it is safe to assume, found indications of arsenic. Near to midnight he made his way to Bishop Auckland, to the police station, and told Superintendent John Henderson.

The following day, Thursday, 18th July, 1872, the superintendent with two sergeants, one of them Hutchinson, went to the Front Street house with a warrant charging Mary Ann with the murder of Charles Edward Cotton. Mrs Dodds had not had time to hand her the money for the clothes and the pawn tickets. It is said that Mary Ann made no reply when Henderson read out the warrant. One would have expected a denial, as she afterwards maintained throughout that she was not guilty. But she could have been overawed, with justification, by the law in action against her, and the police might have been in no mind to listen to her. There is no record of her saying anything as they, with Dr. Kilburn, searched the house. They took away a little powder, some pills, arrowroot, and powdered red lead: a disappointing haul.

Mary Ann was taken to Bishop Auckland and put in a cell in the police station in Bondgate. She appeared in the justice room upstairs the following morning and was remanded in custody. In that morning's *Newcastle Journal*, before she had appeared in court, a report said that there had been dissatisfaction in more than one quarter at the result of the inquest and that it was being said that three of her husbands had died suspiciously when they were insured.

That day, 19th July, the Clerk to the Justices at Bishop Auckland, William Dale Trotter, wrote to the Home Office, to the Secretary of State, asking for an order for exhumation of the body of Charles Edward and analysis of the stomach viscera and other organs and their contents. This was granted and sanctioned. Trotter said that from a post-mortem examination and the evidence of the medical man it appeared that the child had died from natural causes and the jury returned a verdict accordingly. Since the inquest a suspicion had arisen that the child had been poisoned and great excitement had prevailed in the neighbourhood. The child had lived with its stepmother and the suspicion had very naturally been directed against her.

The magistrates had instituted an inquiry through the police, and a statement taken by Superintendent Henderson, which told of previous deaths, and the evidence taken at the inquest were forwarded.

A week later, 26th July, Charles Edward's coffin was dug up before the doctors, Kilburn and Chalmers, and policemen, Henderson and Hutchinson. In an empty house nearby, Kilburn put the viscera in clean bottles which he corked, sealed, labelled, numbered and signed. The stomach which had been dug up from Kilburn's garden was bottled, too. Of the stomach contents Kilburn bottled only nine drachms – just more than a fluid ounce. These bottles, together with faeces passed by the boy shortly before he died, and the items taken from Mary Ann's house, were taken by Sergeant Hutchinson to Dr Thomas Scattergood, lecturer on forensic medicine and toxicology at Leeds School of Medicine. He found arsenic in the contents and substance of both stomach and bowels, and in the liver, lungs, heart, kidneys and in the faeces.

CHAPTER TWO

The first hearing:

August, 1872

Mary Ann was taken to Durham gaol before that first exhumation: she was to spend far longer there than at her last West Auckland home. She must have been held at Bishop Auckland for only a night or two. The old police station and courts in Bondgate are now a deserted, decaying building, labyrinthine, with some of the many rooms in deep darkness even during the day; light comes into the two adjoining cells from a small squarish pane in each, recessed high up in the thick wall. Each cell has a long wooden bed stretching along one side, for two people lying feet to feet. Each half slopes to the middle with a wooden pillow at the top end. Plank beds were introduced into English prisons in 1865, following their use in military prisons. Mattresses, in the main, but not altogether, were then dispensed with. Outside, the section of the enclosed yard at the other side of the cells is penned-in by iron railings.

The committal hearings were held upstairs in a fine, high-ceilinged room. On Wednesday, 21st August, 1872, nearly five weeks after being taken into custody, Mary Ann faced a charge of wilful murder of her seven-year-old stepson, Charles Edward Cotton, by administering arsenic or causing it to be administered. There were two magistrates: the Revd James Hick and J. Jobson. She was said to have had a self-possessed air throughout, but the further detail, that she held a white handkerchief to one side of her face for most of the time does not seem to confirm this.

Old Mrs Dodds gave evidence. She said that on Monday, 8th July, when she was helping Mrs Cotton with the washing, Mrs Cotton told her that Charlie had taken ill the day before and that she could go up and see him if she wanted to. The boy had been asleep, but the next day he was awake and when she asked him if he felt any better he didn't answer. On the Wednesday he seemed to be quite ill, and she had said to Mrs

Cotton: 'I don't think he'll be long here if he keeps at this.' Mrs Cotton hadn't said anything. On the Friday Mrs Cotton had sent for her with the news that the boy was dead. The fits had come on about midnight and he had died shortly before six in the morning. He was lying on a sofa. Usually he slept with Mrs Cotton.

Some six weeks before, when she was helping Mrs Cotton to clean, Mrs Cotton had sent little Charlie to Mr Townend's, the chemist's, for twopennyworth of arsenic and soft soap to rub the bedstead, which, Mrs Cotton said, had bugs in it. The chemist wouldn't serve the boy and Mrs Cotton asked her if she would go for it. This she did, and they used about half the mixture on the bedstead. They didn't find any bugs there, but there were two or three in the mattress. What was left of the mixture was put in an old pint jug and put in the lumber room.

Mrs Dodds said she had once asked Mrs Cotton if it was true that she would have married the excise officer if it wasn't for Charlie. Mrs Cotton had said it wasn't true: Mr Manning liked the boy; he adored the ground he walked on.

After Thomas Riley had told of his conversation with Mary Ann when he had tried to engage her to look after a smallpox patient, the hearing was adjourned – perhaps because Dr Kilburn could not attend. The doctor gave evidence first at the resumed hearing on the Friday. Before a crowded court he said he had seen the boy for the last time on the evening before he died: he had looked pale and waxy and he was suffering from vomiting, purging and pains in the stomach. Mrs Cotton had herself come to his house, leaving a message that the boy was worse. He had seen the boy earlier that day and sent him medicine: ammonia in a state of effervescence. The boy had vomited this. After the early evening visit he gave him a mixture of bismuth, hydrocyanic acid and powders containing an eighth of a grain of morphia.

The post-mortem examination was made early on the Saturday afternoon, thirty-two hours after death. The external appearance was of emaciation. He had not noticed any marks of external violence. The lungs were adherent to the walls of the chest, an indication of a long-standing inflammation. He examined the stomach, a dark brownish red in colour, with a small microscope, and saw two or three particles of white powder which he took to be a portion of the last powder he had given. He had formed his opinion that the child had died from natural causes, chiefly on the ground that many medical authors stated that the post-mortem action of the gastric juices could produce such an appearance. He had not had time to make an analysis of the contents of the stomach; he put these in a jar, which, together with the stomach and some of the intestines, he took home. His further examination on the Wednesday was because of what he had heard.

This remark of Kilburn's reveals how near Mary Ann was to escaping. With no coroner's or jury's request for a chemical analysis, but for the persistence of local feeling and supposition the parts buried in the garden could have been forgotten and the stomach contents eventually thrown out. Kilburn obviously had no suspicions of Mary Ann. He seems to have been on the slow side to begin the chemical examination. He would not want to be presented with evidence pointing to a woman he knew as a murderess; one gathers he was a man who would shrink from the prospect of publicity and of court appearances; and also, if the poison were found, there would be full public revelation of his professional limitations, of his naivety, of how he had been deceived. He was about forty years old at the time. I have been told there was a marriage link between the Rileys and Kilburns. Later it was said it was Riley's insistence more than anything which brought Mary Ann to trial. This link could have been crucial in causing Kilburn to continue the examination.

Archibald Chalmers, surgeon, also gave evidence that Friday. He had seen the boy three times during the week; the last time he was considerably weaker. So, there had been a minimum of five visits from the doctors. It was no out-of-sight killing but sleight-of-hand before experts, who, it is true, were not expecting a trick. A defender of Mary Ann, however, could maintain that this points to her innocence.

The evidence from Dr Scattergood from Leeds was damning. He was forthright and certain. There was no appearances of enteric or gastric fever. The stomach and upper portion of the smaller bowel showed marks of inflammation caused, Scattergood said, by an irritant poison. There was evidence of blood. In the stomach contents there was more than half a grain of white arsenic or arsenious acid. Death, in his opinion, was from poisoning by arsenic. He said none of the articles taken from Mary Ann's house contained arsenic: the powder had been borax and a little morphia; the pills, vegetable material, had probably come from a herbalist.

Hick asked Mary Ann if she had anything to say. She said,

'No,' in a low voice, and was committed for trial at the next Durham Assizes.

So again Mary Ann Cotton was taken down Bondgate and down the length of Newgate Street to the railway station and the ten miles by train to Durham, and then twice across the looping River Wear to the county gaol at the head of Old Elvet – confirmed as the end of her wandering. Once for certain in the summer of 1872, either on this occasion or after one of her remand appearances, she was walked from the court to the Bishop Auckland railway-station flanked by two tall policemen who made her look small. On that walk some people hurried ahead, letting others know that she was coming, and some mothers ran out to hide their children from her. Her name was used to conjure up a bogey woman to frighten children into obedience. The children reacted by making-up play rhymes. She wore a black and white shawl over her black dress on that walk. Such shawls, fashionable at the time, ceased to be so in that Durham area.

After the hearing, the *Durham County Advertiser* said that other deaths in her house, in which she was alleged to have had a pecuniary interest, would also be investigated. They said there was talk of exhuming the body of Nattrass.

Nearly a fortnight later, on 5th September, Trotter wrote to the Home Secretary that the justices were of the opinion that it was necessary for the ends of justice to have Joseph Nattrass's body exhumed. Nattrass, he said, was ill for a very short time and died shortly after making his will in favour of Mrs Cotton. The body of Nattrass was dug up on Saturday morning, 14th September. It had been buried in new ground to the north of St Helen's Auckland church for five and a half months and the digging party was led by the sexton to various plots – seven were opened – before the right one was found. Riley volunteered to affirm in court that the body was indeed that of Nattrass. Kilburn, assisted by a Dr Easby of Darlington, carried out the examination in a farm outhouse.

On 25th September Trotter wrote again to the Home Office quoting the unequivocal Scattergood: 'There is no doubt that Nattrass was poisoned by arsenic. I find there is a considerable quantity in the stomach and bowels, between four and five grains of it being still in the state of undissolved powder. Arsenic is in all the viscera.'

Trotter was directed by the magistrates to ask for authority to exhume three more bodies, especially those of the other two

Cotton children. The other one was that of Frederick Cotton, the father. The order was granted and analysis sanctioned by return of post, but the exhumation was postponed because of the information coming to light from the police enquiries into Mary Ann's life before she came to West Auckland, and on 1st October Superintendent Henderson sent a report to the Home Office.

This said that Mary Ann was born about 1832, and that her father, Michael Robson, was killed in 1846. She married William Mowbray, a labourer at Murton Colliery in County Durham. They moved to the Plymouth area. When they returned five years later she said she had had four children and all had died. Mowbray got work at South Hetton and a fifth child of theirs died. They moved to Hendon, Sunderland, and in a nine-month spell there, two children and Mowbray himself died. All were insured with the British and Prudential company. Mary Ann then worked as a nurse at the old infirmary in Sunderland and married George Ward after his discharge as a patient. Ward soon died, rather suspiciously, at the age of thirty-three.

She became housekeeper to James Robinson, a widower and shipyard foreman at Pallion, Sunderland. They married six months later, but before that three of his children had died, as well as her remaining child by Mowbray, a girl of nine. Later her first child by Robinson died. Robinson forbade her to insure his life; they had a row when she ran him into debt, and she left him. Robinson now was convinced that she had poisoned the children.

Twelve of the deaths were from gastric fever with symptoms resembling those of arsenic poisoning. By the names of two of Robinson's children and her own nine-year-old girl, Henderson had marked asterisks denoting particularly strong suspicions of poisoning.

Trotter asked if it was not now desirable to exhume some of the bodies buried in Sunderland, especially those of the three children, rather than the three at West Auckland. The Home Office minute stated that the case was very serious and that an application for a licence would be entertained, but the bodies had been long interred and the justices should be satisfied that exhumation was necessary.

They decided not to do anything about the Sunderland burials for the time being and on 15th October a party of at least eight medical men, headed by Kilburn, arrived at the St Helen's Auckland graveyard. Thomas Riley, too, was there. They had to be content with the bodies of the two children as that of Frederick Cotton, buried thirteen months before, could not be found. Sergeant Hutchinson's party of labourers began digging at five in the morning. None of the graves was numbered or marked and although the memory of the seventy-two-year-old sexton, Joseph Drummond, operated well in finding the graves of the children – only two other plots were opened – it failed time after time with that of Frederick Cotton. A report of the day says the graves were 'as thick and close as furrows in a lea field'. Care had to be taken in clearing the coffin lids in case the yellow-painted names were made illegible. Two days later some of the people present at Cotton's burial had their say about the position of the grave, at least twelve more were opened without finding his.

Four days earlier, after two exhumations and committal proceedings in one case, the *Durham Chronicle* printed the police report to the Home Office, with extra detail, in two wide columns headed, 'The Great Poisoning Case at West Auckland: Horrible Revelations'. They said the report showed a series of suspected crimes almost without parallel in the country. Mary Ann Cotton, who had a degree of intelligence not often found in women of her class, was suspected of being responsible for no fewer than twenty deaths: those of her mother, three husbands, fifteen children and a lodger. Between her marriages to Robinson and Cotton, it was said, she appeared to have led a loose life.

The *Durham Chronicle* article included a reprint of one which had appeared in the *Sunderland Times*, based on an interview with Robinson. In this Robinson said he had advertised for a housekeeper when his wife died. Mary Ann applied and seemed to be a suitable person. He had thought she possessed all the domestic qualities a husband could desire in a wife and he resolved to marry her.

A Durham city resident, Mr H. I. Marshall, forwarded a copy of the *Durham Chronicle* to the Home Secretary, Henry Austin Bruce, on the grounds that a person charged should not be prejudiced before trial. The Home Office minute said, 'The Secretary of State cannot prevent the publication of such paragraphs.'

A month later, on 11th November, Trotter was ready to go ahead with the other three cases and he applied to the Home Office for a writ of habeas corpus to bring Mary Ann from Durham on as many days as might be found necessary, in order that witnesses might be examined in her presence. He was told that the Home Secretary had no power to do this; application must be made to a judge.

The application was not made because of Mary Ann's condition. Her baby was now due in less than two months, and Trotter forwarded a certificate to the Home Office from William Boyd, the surgeon at the prison. Dated 22nd November, 1872, this read : 'I certify that Mary Ann Cotton a prisoner in Durham Gaol is in her seventh month of pregnancy. She is in such a state of health as would allow her to be removed to Bishop Auckland, but for her condition it is uncertain how long such may continue.'

In his letter Trotter said analysis had shown that young Frederick Cotton and the baby had also died from arsenical poisoning. As Mrs Cotton was now very considerably advanced in pregnancy it was desirable to have the trial postponed to the spring assizes. Would the Treasury allow the expense of an application to a judge for such a postponement? Also would the Treasury pay for an application for a writ of habeas corpus, although they might not be able to make use of such a writ just now?

The Home Office minute to the Secretary assumed that these necessary expenses would be allowed. Bruce thought this would be so, but advised having a word with the Exchequer of Civil Law Accounts before telling Trotter. The department in Spring Gardens replied that in every case expenses in bringing a prisoner before a magistrate devolved upon local funds, and they suggested that the examination should take place at the gaol which would make a writ unnecessary. Bruce said he did not see how the proceedings could very well take place at the gaol. He advised that the expenses of the writ should be borne by local funds, but that the cost of an application to a court for postponement of the trial would be allowed.

While these niceties of accounting were being sorted out in London, Mary Ann had no money to hire professional advice. There was some local concern about her lack of defence. Later she was to write bitterly about the little advice she received. Charles Chapman, a young solicitor in Market Place, Durham, first undertook to act for her, through George F. Smith, of Gibbon Street, Bishop Auckland. Smith is described as clerk to Chapman. When Chapman heard there could be other grave charges he thought the case too big and serious for him, and with Smith he saw Mary Ann in Durham and told her she needed a more experienced attorney. He disliked having his name associated with hers and in a letter to the *Durham County Advertiser* on 27th November he said that Mary Ann had signed a paper releasing him and had said she would like Smith to conduct her defence. The two men saw Mary Ann in Durham prison on 26th July, the day when Charles Edward's body was being exhumed and when she had been in custody for a week. Chapman then witnessed an authorization by her for Smith to take possession and dispose of her furniture.

Lowrey had taken a fair amount of her belongings with the intention of buying them himself or selling them for her. Writing to her on 22nd February, 1873, he said,

> Mr Smith come to me about the 26 of August and said you give him power to sell all your furniture he said you have something you bought from her I said yes he said you must give up what you dont want I done so I give him the Bed the Carpets Knives forks Box and some more little thing so what I kept come to £3. 19. 6 and what I give you and him and expenses there is 7 shillings due yet he took all your things to Bishop Auckland sold them for £13 he did not sell any off your garments as fare as I know that day he come he had a paper singed by you and the key off your house he from the Police at BP Auckland If all be well I will be at Durham.

Lowrey must have told her these details before, as he says,

> I must say that it make me look very simple for to write on one subject so often – but as you say you lost the letter I will tell you once more.

His peevish letter begins abruptly; 'Mrs Cotton,' and ends, 'So this is all that I know if Mr Smith has done rong more is the pitty

I am yours respectfully
Lowrey.'

After seeing Lowrey, Smith went to Mrs Dodds and demanded and got from her the pawn tickets. Mary Ann had lent Quick-Manning a silver watch (Nattrass left her his watch in his will), and Smith went to Quick-Manning and got it. The fact that Mary Ann must have told Smith this is indicative of her acceptance of the end of that affair.

With this money raised from Mary Ann's possessions Smith did very little indeed. He said he gave a watching brief to a barrister for the first short day of the magistrates' hearing at Bishop Auckland on 21st August and that this had absorbed the lot.

With less than forty-eight hours to live, Mary Ann wrote again to Lowrey, who, on behalf of the foster-mother who took the child, had enquired about the clothes which had been pawned.

> March th 22, 1873.
>
> My der frend,
>
> I did not give Mistr Smith Authority to get the pawn tickets from Mary Ann Dodds. I did not know he had got them till Hutchinson at Bishop Auckland told me.
>
> Mary Ann Cotton.
>
> Witness: Mary Douglas, Schoolmistress, County Gaol, Durham.

The thought of Smith exasperated her to the end. She wrote to a neighbour,

> Smith had lead me rong. He told me not to speake A single Worde if i Was Asked Ever so hard or Ever so mutch, i Was not to say it was Wrong, that Would be All don in durham. He has never brote forth Won Witness fore me, he new What they Ware Wanted fore, not only the childe, but for mysealfe. I do not Want nothing but the trouth of Every Won then ie Would have A Chance fore my Life . . . if it had not been for smith I should make 5 or 6 of them stand With thar toungs tyde.

The absence of a defender at the further committal hearings at Bishop Auckland in February was deplored by the prosecution.

On 10th January, 1873, Mary Ann gave birth to her last child, her twelfth, a girl, in Durham Gaol. The child was christened Margaret Edith Quick-Manning Cotton.

On 7th February, Trotter wrote to the Home Secretary asking if the treasury would take up the prosecution in all four cases. He said there was every reason to believe that Mary Ann had been a wholesale poisoner. The Treasury had undertaken prosecutions of a similar nature, and it seemed very important that they should do so in these cases, the more especially as the scale of allowances in prosecutions was now so low that it was with extreme difficulty that any attorney of sufficient capability and standing could be got to undertake them, and it was certain that none would undertake to do justice to cases of the intricacies and importance of these, on the usual scale of assize costs. Mrs Cotton had quite recovered from the effects of her confinement and the three remaining cases were ready for investigation before the justices whenever a habeas corpus was obtained, and the justices hoped the Treasury would at once obtain this.

Bruce agreed immediately that the Treasury should prosecute, and in a letter from the Home Office on 10th February the Solicitor to the Treasury was instructed to take charge. Bruce also said that if Trotter was advised to do so he could proceed to the investigation of other cases against Mary Ann. So the writ of habeas corpus was eventually obtained by the Treasury's solicitor and a fortnight after his request Trotter prosecuted at Bishop Auckland on behalf of the Treasury on the three further charges.

There was no defence at all against his case. Mary Ann wrote to a Newcastle lawyer in Eldon Square and received an impersonal reply, dated 12th February, 1873.

> Mr Blackwell duly received Mrs Cotton's letter. He has been retained by Mr Smith, acting for Mr Chapman, Solicitor, Durham, to defend her at the ensuing Assizes but regrets that up to this time has not received any instructions from either of the above named gentlemen.

A few days later Smith wrote to her from Bishop Auckland.

> Madam,
> You will be brought over here on Friday first on the other Cases when I will see you. I wrote Mr Blackwell the other day about the Case.
> Yours truly
> Geo. F. Smith.

Smith never gave Blackwell instructions, and he, himself, was not even present on Mary Ann's behalf at the Bishop Auckland proceedings.

CHAPTER THREE

Three more at Bishop Auckland:

February, 1873

When I am dead and coffined, put my glengarry cap on my head

Early on Friday, 21st February, Mary Ann was taken by cab from the county gaol to Durham railway station for the 8.28 train to Bishop Auckland. She carried her six-week-old baby in her arms, and was in charge of the head warder, Thompson Smith, and the matron, Mrs Margaret Robinson. She had been seven months in prison and the law now leapt into gear for a fast final run.

People wanted to gaze at her. They assembled at Durham station, at stations en route and at Bishop Auckland they lined the streets. Thompson Smith waited until the bulk of the passengers had got clear of the platform before he gave the word for them to leave the train and the matron took the baby for a time with Mary Ann holding on to her arm.

The magistrates were Colonel Hall of Heighington, the chairman, and J. Jobson, Major Hodgson and the Revd J. W. Hick. Two rows of chairs were provided for chosen ladies and gentlemen, others stood: all had received tickets from Trotter. Mary Ann was given a seat facing the elderly magistrates. She and the matron shared the nursing of the baby. Mary Ann breast-fed the child who, in the main, was quiet and caused little distraction. It was in a black and white checked shawl and the pink lace which trimmed the satin cap was the only touch of colour about mother and child. Mary Ann wore a black cotton dress, her black and white checked shawl and a black bonnet trimmed with crepe. The top of her dark hair, brushed back, was enclosed in a net. Her face was pale and clear and her expression intent.

Many of the reporters – there were sixteen there, including two from Leeds and four from Newcastle – commented on her appealing looks: one contrasted her delicate and prepossessing appearance with the deliberate coarsening of portraits of her. She had lost colour and weight since August.

The charge of the wilful murder of Joseph Nattrass, aged thirty-five, on Easter Monday, 1st April, 1872, was taken first.

Trotter said that of Mary Ann's four husbands, three were dead. She had married once when a husband was alive. She took in lodgers and after the death of her last husband, Frederick Cotton, Nattrass, a pitman, lodged with her. About a fortnight before he died he complained to fellow-workmen of wanting to be sick. he had to take to his bed, where he was treated for gastric fever by Dr Richardson. The evidence about who administered the poison was of a circumstantial character, but Trotter said that he would show that Mrs Cotton was the only person who attended Nattrass; that when neighbours suggested he was not being given sufficient food she put them off, never allowing one of them to give him anything; and that she was in possession of arsenic. She had said that the body of her baby should be held back for burial until Nattrass died; she sent out for stockings and things to lay-out Nattrass before he was dead, and she received Nattrass's burial money a few days after his death.

George Vickers said Nattrass and he were marrows at West Auckland Colliery and that Nattrass, after three days of being unwell, looked very ill on the last shift they wrought together.

Thomas Hall, an overman, said he had known Nattrass for fifteen or sixteen years and he was a pretty healthy man. He saw him on the Sunday, the day before he died, in an upstairs room in the prisoner's house, and the prisoner contrived to stay in the room all the time he was there. There was a dead child in the house and he asked her why she didn't have it buried. She had said she didn't intend to yet as she thought Nattrass wouldn't live long – meaning that they could be buried together.

Mary Ann declined to ask any questions.

Phoebe Robson, a pitman's wife, often in Mary Ann's house, said the baby died on the Thursday and was buried on Easter Sunday. Nattrass was bad in the bowels and sick: the prisoner never left his bedside and wouldn't let anyone else be about him. Witness herself, had suggested many times that Nattrass should have some food, but Mrs Cotton had said he couldn't take anything. He had fits, particularly towards the end, and

Mrs Cotton would hold him down, otherwise he would have come out of bed. He would clench his hands together, grind his teeth, turn up the whites of his eyes and draw his legs up. She hadn't thought there was much the matter with him until he began to take the fits. When they were mentioned to the doctor, the doctor said he didn't understand them. When the child died her sister-in-law, Sarah Smith, asked Mrs Cotton if she would have it buried on the Saturday, but she said she would wait till the Sunday. On the Sunday she said she would let it be as Nattrass was not going to live long and she would have them buried together.

Again Mary Ann declined to question, although an obvious point to have made clear was that the baby was buried later on the Sunday, 31st March. Nattrass died the following day and was not buried until the Wednesday, 3rd April.

Sarah Smith, aged forty-three, a neighbour in Johnson Terrace, said she was often in the house during Nattrass's illness. He complained of his stomach and bowels especially when he was having fits. When he had these he clashed his head against the wall and bedpost, and he bent back his toes as if he were in cramp. He generally turned on his side. When the fit was over he said it was a bad one, or not a very bad one, as the case might be. She had asked if she could give him beef tea or anything but Mrs Cotton had said not. Nattrass didn't say much really but he complained of thirst. She saw Mrs Cotton twice give him a cup of tea. She had two small teapots on a table nearby. She was there on the Friday when Mrs Cotton told Dr Richardson that Nattrass had had a bad night with fits. The doctor said: 'Fits! What kind of fits are they? It's very strange he's always taking fits when I'm not here.'

On the Saturday little Charlie Cotton brought in a pair of men's white stockings. These didn't seem to suit the prisoner who said if anything should happen to Nattrass she hadn't a pair that would do for him. On the Monday that Nattrass died Mrs Cotton said she had sent for a woman called Tate to wash some linen, but the woman couldn't come. She said the linen used to lay-out the child needed to be washed to lay-out Nattrass.

Jane Hedley, aged twenty-four, wife of George Hedley, a miner, also of Johnson Terrace, said she was in the house when Dr Richardson called. Nattrass said the pain hadn't left him, and the doctor said if he could stop the purging he thought he would get better. The doctor said Nattrass had a fever, and when Nattrass said he knew better than that, Dr Richardson said then it was no use his coming. Nattrass said he hadn't taken the doctor's medicine. She was there when Nattrass died in a fit. Mrs Cotton was holding him down. She had seen Mrs Cotton give him something to drink several times, but never any food. On the Thursday Mrs Cotton told her that Nattrass wanted her, Mrs Cotton, to have his watch and club money and that he had said that she had been his best friend. A week after Nattrass's death Mrs Cotton was in her house, about half a dozen doors away, helping her to clean. Mrs Cotton asked her to go to her house for a pot on the pantry shelf which had soft soap and arsenic in it. She had got this, she said, to clean her beds with. She went for it and Mrs Cotton put a little on the wall, about a knife-pointful. There were about two tablespoonfuls in the pot. Mrs Cotton just left the pot in her house; she didn't take it back.

Elijah Atkinson, aged forty-four, a Cleveland countryman and now a pointsman, said he was sent for on the Thursday. He asked Nattrass specially if it was his desire that Mrs Cotton should have the whole of his effects. Nattrass said it was, as he had no friend that had looked to him. He had made a will; Nattrass made his mark to it, and he and George Hedley witnessed it. He gave the will to Mrs Cotton, who was in the room the whole time it was being made out. Nattrass had ten pounds in the Oddfellows Club, held at the Dun Cow, Shildon, as well as his watch hanging at the bedhead and his clothes.

Evidence was given of £10. 15s. being paid out by the Oddfellows Club, called the Rose of Shildon Lodge. Fifteen shillings was for nine days' sick pay. Five pounds was handed to George Hedley when he went to the lodge with the death certificate and a note from Mrs Cotton. The rest was paid direct to Mrs Cotton. No receipts were given, as they were not customary.

Thomas Charlton Richardson, surgeon and physician, of Lanchester Terrace, West Auckland, said he thought it was Mrs Cotton who called and wanted him to attend to Nattrass. She described the symptoms and without seeing Nattrass he prescribed a grain of morphia and an effervescent mixture. The first time he saw Nattrass was on the Tuesday before he died. There was much irritability of the bowels and the bladder, but this was an old complaint. He gave him an astringent mixture and more morphia, which gave relief. On the Wednesday he was told Nattrass had had a fit, but Nattrass said he didn't remember it. He sent some bi-carbonate of soda and hydrocyanic and carbonate of lithia. He changed the medicine for the last time on the Thursday, when he sent morphia and acetate of lead. Nattrass always said he was very much relieved. It was the neighbours who continually said how bad he had been. The symptoms of irritability remained, but on the last two days he thought Nattrass was getting better and would recover. Nattrass never complained about having a fit. He couldn't believe he had them: he couldn't see anything to account for them. He considered the complaint to be inflammation of the mucous membrane of the bowels and high irritability of the neck of the bladder. The symptoms were consistent with arsenical poisoning. There was no arsenic in anything he had prescribed.

Dr Kilburn spoke of the exhumation of the body, identified by Thomas Riley and easily recognisable by the shape of the forehead and colour of the hair. The forehead was lofty and had a peculiar square shape. He had put the parts in clean, mostly new, untainted bottles; the stomach had been placed between two inverted soup-plates; these and a sample of adjacent soil had been taken by Sergeant Hutchinson to Dr Scattergood.

Scattergood said over three-fifths of the stomach surface was intensely inflamed, and its deep red colour was in strong contrast to the natural pale colour of the rest. The duodenum, the part of the small intestine next to the stomach, was also highly inflamed, and so was the rectum which was bright red. There were none of the appearances of gastric fever. He found arsenic in the stomach and bowels, in the liver, lungs, heart, kidney and spleen. The arsenic in the bowels amounted to seventeen and three-quarter grains, about four grains being solid. The earth of the graveyard had contained no arsenic. He had no doubt but that Nattrass died from poisoning by arsenic: he added that he gave that opinion with very great confidence.

TROTTER: 'Have you formed any opinion as to whether death resulted from one dose or repeated doses?'

SCATTERGOOD: 'I could not speak to that.'

Mary Ann who had listened attentively and not shown any agitation was then asked if she had anything to say to the charge.

'I have nothing to say at present.'

COLONEL HALL: 'Then you will be committed to take your trial at the ensuing Durham Assizes for the wilful murder of

Joseph Nattrass . . . Do you wish to have witnesses bound over to attend on your behalf?'

'I have some witnesses.'

'Are there any here?'

'There are three here.'

'Do you wish to have them bound over for your defence?'

'Yes.'

'Do you wish to call them now?'

'No.'

SUPERINTENDENT HENDERSON: 'What are their names?'

'Jane Hedley, George Hedley and Eliza Atkinson.'

HENDERSON: 'They are witnesses for the prosecution.'

TROTTER: 'It becomes a question whether we can bind them over if they are not examined.'

HALL: 'Are we to understand you to say you do not wish to call witnesses at present for your defence?'

'No, sir.'

The magistrates deliberated with Trotter, who said Mary Ann must call witnesses now if she wished them to be bound over. She said she did not wish to call the witnesses at present.

Trotter then opened the other two cases by recalling Jane Hedley – one of the witnesses Mary Ann had hoped to have in her defence – and asking her questions about the deaths of the two children. He did this now, he said, because of the state of Mrs Hedley's health. After her evidence the examinations were adjourned until the following Tuesday and Mary Ann was taken back to Durham by the 6.15 train. Superintendent and Mrs Henderson provided her with a midday dinner at the Sun Inn, Bishop Auckland.

In spite of a snowstorm on the Tuesday people still came out to try to see her. She was again escorted by the chief warder and matron, and carried her baby. That trip to Bishop Auckland gave her her last look at countryside, villages and streets – all snow-covered.

In court, Trotter said Mrs Cotton had stated that a person named Smith, who had sold her furniture and other things by her authority for the purpose of her defence, was not to be found; and that she now had no more money.

Major Hodgson said he had just seen Smith in the street.

Thompson Smith, the warder, told the court that Smith had received about twenty pounds from Mrs Cotton. She had been surprised he was not present on her behalf last Friday although she had made no complaint. Smith had been in court on a former occasion and taken notes. She had written to him but had received no reply.

Trotter said that as far as the Crown was concerned they would much rather that the prisoner was defended. They wished her to have all the assistance possible. It was a great disadvantage not having someone to defend her now. There were many points of evidence which might be got up in her defence.

Colonel Hall said that if Smith had got money from Mrs Cotton it was only right that she should have benefit from it. Trotter suggested that Smith should be called to account. He said a letter had come to him from a Stockton man, a Mr Charles Murray, saying that if friends of Mrs Cotton would communicate with him he would find able counsel for her at Durham assizes. The letter was handed to Mary Ann.

Colonel Hall asked if Mrs Cotton was aware that at the assizes she was sure to have counsel assigned to her by the Crown. Thompson Smith said she had been told that this was usual in such cases.

Later that day George Smith was brought into court. He said it was perfectly true that the prisoner had supplied him with money for the purpose of having the case watched for her, but that was for the first case and counsel had been retained in it. It was not so in this case.

Chapman and Smith made a deplorable pair – one scared and squeamish, the other conscienceless, concerned only with making what little money he could. They were foolish, too: others would have seized the opportunity of defending Mary Ann against the circumstantial evidence and made a name for themselves. Smith did not get away with things completely: the disapproval voiced by the magistrates was taken up later by the press. Smith in effect worked against Mary Ann. He would not get out of the way and make room for others and no one had the interest and resolve to circumvent him. He was there, holding, obstructing, doing nothing positive. He advised Mary Ann not to speak; he made no effort to assemble a defence; he took useless notes at the August hearing, and one doubts whether he had to pay counsel anything.

The first case on the Tuesday was that of young Frederick Cotton. From the limited record of what he did and said, this ten-year-old seems to have been a likeable lad – polite, sensitive, trusting, imaginative. But, his parents gone, he made no impression on the feelings of the woman he had to accept as substitute. She probably was engrossed in her affair with Quick-Manning about the time of the boy's death.

Jane Hedley's evidence had been that Mary Ann had never left the boy: that she had seen her give him drinks from a little teapot, but no food. He had died at five minutes to twelve on Sunday night, 10th March. In the afternoon he asked for his cap and he had it on when he was laid out and put in his coffin.

The first witness on the Tuesday, Sarah Smith, said that early in the week of the boy's illness, Mrs Cotton came and asked her to have a look at him, saying he had a pain in the bowels but really he was bad all over. He was then lying on a sofa and trying to be sick. Mrs Cotton said she was hoping he hadn't got smallpox as she'd been nursing patients and people would talk so. The next day the boy was worse and in bed and Mrs Cotton was trying to stop the bleeding from a leech-wound on the right side of his bowels. He was now being sick, and he complained of thirst. Mrs Cotton gave him drinks out of a teapot and these often made him vomit. She used two teapots. Dr Kilburn's assistant came and stopped the bleeding. The boy was sick so often that sometimes he couldn't get his head to the basin. She saw Mrs Cotton try to give him tea and toast once, but he couldn't take it. The night before he died he wanted someone to pray with him and she had gone for Elijah Atkinson. On the Sunday afternoon the boy asked for his black glengarry cap. Mrs Cotton passed it to her and she gave it to the boy who put it on and asked her if it was all right. He said that when he was dead and coffined he was to have his glengarry cap on, that he was to be buried in it. When they were coffining him she asked Mrs Cotton if it was all right putting the cap on the boy and she said, yes, all that he desired should be done. So she, Sarah Smith, had put the cap on the boy. When he was laid-out Mrs Cotton said they all had to have a cup of tea and a piece of fruit loaf. Jane Hedley had brought in the loaf the night before.

Jane Hedley, there after all on the Tuesday and recalled again, said that on the Saturday night, when Mrs Cotton heard that she was going into Bishop Auckland, she asked her to bring back one of the best spice loaves.

Phoebe Robson said Mrs Cotton told her that the boy had the gastric fever. Mrs Cotton generally used two little teapots; one stood on the bed-head and the other on the chimney-piece.

Elizabeth Atkinson, aged forty-nine, wife of Elijah Atkinson, lived two doors from Mary Ann in Johnson Terrace. On the Wednesday she had asked the boy if he could take anything. He was with his stepmother and he didn't reply, but he asked if he could see Mr Atkinson.

'Yes. Why?' she had asked.

'Because I want him to pray with me,' Frederick said. (Sarah Smith said he asked for Elijah Atkinson also on the Saturday.)

Back home she had prepared some rice and milk and sent it in with the girl. She next saw the boy on the Saturday when Mrs Cotton, sitting at the bedside, said he had had a restless night. She asked him again if he could take anything and this time he said he could, so she went back and prepared some beef tea and took it up herself. Mrs Cotton was still at the bedside. The boy said, 'Thank you, Mrs Atkinson.' Then suddenly Mrs Cotton said the boy was not to have it. She had been surprised and hurt, and Mrs Cotton muttered that Frederick couldn't take anything and that it would do him no good. And she had said, 'Well, Mrs Cotton, it *is* a very untimely hour to take beef tea,' and she had turned away, grieved, and come out. Mrs Cotton used to give the boy drinks out of two teapots, the larger black, the other brown. She said it was easier to drink from them.

Dr Chalmers, who lived at Evenwood, two miles south-west of West Auckland, said he made up the medicine which Dr Kilburn prescribed. There was no arsenic in it. He thought the boy had gastric fever and that the medicine should have brought him some relief, but it had no effect whatever.

Dr Kilburn said he saw the boy first on Monday, 4th March, when the boy complained of pain in the bowels: this was increased by pressure. There was some thirst; the tongue was dry and glazed, and there was anxiety of countenance. He treated him for enteric fever. Leeches were applied and he prescribed a mixture of bismuth, bi-carbonate of potass and a few minims of hydrocyanic acid. He saw the boy again on the Wednesday; the sickness and purging continued, and he ordered a blister to put on the boy's stomach. He attended the boy up to his death on Sunday, 10th March.

He was present at the disinterring of the body on 15th October. The glengarry cap was still on the boy's head. Sergeant Hutchinson took the bottles and plates and a parcel of soil to Leeds and he went there a few days later and examined the parts with Dr Scattergood. He saw no appearances of enteric fever. There was strong evidence of poisoning by arsenic.

Scattergood said the stomach was much inflamed in patches: there were bright red streaks. He found just more than a grain of arsenic in the stomach and bowels, nearly all dissolved or absorbed, and nearly half a grain in the solid organs. The boy had died from poisoning by arsenic.

The next witness seems to have perturbed Mary Ann more than any other, and he was the only one she questioned. Thomas Detchon, an assistant with William Owen, a chemist, of Collingwood Street, Newcastle, said he remembered perfectly a woman coming into the shop in January, 1869, as asking for threepennyworth of soft soap and arsenic. She said she wanted it for cleaning bedsteads and for destroying bugs. She gave the name of Mary Ann Booth. He had picked Mary Ann out of a dozen women in Durham gaol and he was positive she was the woman who came into the shop. (In January, 1869, Mary Ann was married to James Robinson and living at Pallion, Sunderland, some thirteen miles from Newcastle. Five children in the Robinson household had died during the previous two years.)

Detchon said he told the woman he could not sell the arsenic without a witness, and he had recommended a preparation called 'Bugs Specific'. The woman said she would rather have the other and left; then she returned with another woman who gave the name of Elizabeth Robson. (Robson was Mary Ann's maiden name.) Detchon produced the poison book with its entry: 'Jan. 21st, 1869. Mary Ann Booth, purchased threepennyworth of arsenic and soft soap, for destroying bugs. Elizabeth Robson, witness.' The mixture comprised an ounce of arsenic and an ounce and a half of soft soap.

Major Hodgson asked how much the 'Bugs Specific' would have cost, and Detchon said sixpence.

Many Ann then asked her poor question, one about what time of day did he say she had visited the shop? Detchon said: 'To the best of my remembrance it was between two and three in the day when you were there.' 'That will do,' Mary Ann said.

Jane Hedley, recalled yet again, told again of collecting the pot with arsenic and soft soap in it from Mary Ann's home in the first week of April. She was to give the same important evidence in the case of the fourteen-month-old baby later in the day.

The agent for the Prudential Insurance Company, James

Young of Shildon, said Mrs Cotton had insured all three children. He had paid her £5. 15s. on the death of young Frederick.

Mary Ann called no one, and said she had nothing to say.

She was committed for trial at the next assizes.

The case of her own son, the baby, Robert Robson Cotton, who died on Thursday, 28th March, 1872, followed immediately. Jane Hedley's earlier evidence had been that the child began to be ill about a week before he died. He was often sick. 'I saw the child fetch very much,' she said. The two children and Nattrass seemed to have the same kind of symptoms. Mrs Cotton was the only person who attended to the child, and she gave him food at the breast. The child was not weaned.

Sarah Smith said she thought teething had made the child poorly. On the day he died he had seemed to be improving: at dinner-time he had dipped a piece of bread into a jar of syrup and she had said to Mrs Cotton, 'Robbie is all right now,' and Mrs Cotton said he was. When she went back into the house that night Mrs Cotton was kneeling by the cradle upstairs – Nattrass, the lodger, was ill in bed – and the child gave such a heavy fetch and took such a long time to start breathing again and its eyes were so fixed that she thought it was dying.

She said to Mrs Cotton: 'He's dying. Who shall I fetch?' Mrs Cotton said, 'Nobody.'

Sarah Smith said she then asked Mrs Cotton what time the change had taken place, but Mrs Cotton muttered her reply and she couldn't make it out. She asked again who she should get to come in, and Mrs Cotton said she might get the doctor in. When she got back from Dr Kilburn's, Mary Tate and Jane Hedley were in the bedroom and Mary Tate asked her if she had ever seen such a change as this. She said she never had. The child was fetching a heavy fetch again and she asked Mrs Cotton what she had been giving it. Mrs Cotton said, 'Nothing but a teaspoonful of syrup.' Mr Chalmers came and when he was examining the child Mrs Cotton went into a fit, but she soon came out of it. When the doctor had left, Mrs Cotton asked her to take the child out of the cradle, and added if she was frightened she would take it out herself. So she, Sarah Smith, took the child out of the cradle and she had it on her knee for about an hour. It kept fetching, but the intervals got longer. When she had put it back into the cradle she hadn't known if it would have the strength to be sick again. 'But it never fetched any more, it was dead then.' During the time the child was ill

Mrs Cotton attended it well, and she couldn't say she ever saw her give the child anything but the breast.

Mary Tate, a widow, said she had been doing some cleaning in Mary Ann's house. On the day the child died he seemed to be a great deal better. 'At dinner-time the child was standing on its mamma's knee, getting its dinner with us. Mr Chalmers saw it at that time.' She went to her own home about two o'clock, leaving Mrs Cotton alone in the house with the child and Joe Nattrass, who was ill upstairs. When she returned about two hours later the child was very ill. She was astonished and asked Mrs Cotton what was the matter with it. Mrs Cotton said, 'My child, Mrs Tate, is a great deal worse; and don't disturb it.' Mrs Tate then asked if she might go and bring somebody in, but Mrs Cotton said, No, the child was dying, and she hadn't to bring anybody in. But she had been uncomfortable and she left the house and called Sarah Smith in. She went back in the evening and Mrs Cotton took a fit when the child was dying.

Phoebe Robson said the day before the child died Mrs Cotton asked her if she could make a nightdress for him. She did so and took it up on the Thursday night when the child was still alive, but later that night she helped to lay him out in it.

Chalmers said he first saw the child on the Wednesday. He didn't prescribe for him, as he considered him teething and not in any danger. The next day when he saw him, between twelve and one, he was quite well, but when Mrs Smith came for him, between six and seven in the evening, the child was in convulsions. Chalmers said, 'I stayed nearly an hour, and when I left he was dying. The difference which I saw between twelve and six o'clock is not unusual: children sometimes die in teething before a medical man can be brought.'

Dr Kilburn said he was called in on the Tuesday. The child was suffering from a slight febrile attack caused by teething, and he ordered a saline mixture and half a dozen grey powders of mercury and chalk. He saw him again on the Thursday morning – the day the child died – and he seemed to have completely recovered. 'He was prattling on his mother's knee.' He was present at the exhumation. The grave was only a few yards from young Frederick Cotton's. From the appearance of the viscera he considered there was evidence of arsenical poisoning.

Dr Scattergood said about half the inner surface of the stomach was inflamed and of a decidedly red colour. It contained a small quantity of mucous and when diffused in water this deposited a sediment of arsenic. The coats of the stomach, the bowels, and the liver also contained small quantities of arsenic, although the total amount was less than a hundred and twentieth of a grain. There was no disease. Convulsions by teething would not have produced the appearances he saw. His opinion was that death resulted from poisoning by arsenic.

Thomas Detchon, the chemist's assistant, then gave similar evidence to that which he had given in the case of young Frederick Cotton. Colonel Hall, no doubt conscious of the four years which had passed, asked him if he was sure that it was between two and three o'clock when he sold the poison? 'To the best of my recollection,' Detchon said.

'And you never saw her from 1869 until you pointed her out in gaol?' Hall asked.

'No, sir.'

'Had you ever seen her photograph?'

'Yes, I saw it in the early part of November, and I saw the prisoner in the gaol in the latter part of that month.'

'But you swear to the prisoner irrespective of this?'

'Yes, I do.'

Turning to Mary Ann, Colonel Hall said, 'Have you any questions to ask?'

She said, 'I have nothing to ask or say at present.'

She was formally committed to take her trial in this case also, making a fourth charge of wilful murder to be preferred against her.

Was Detchon right or wrong about Mary Ann? With our evidence no one can be sure. As far as is known, 1869 was a poison-free year for her, but a Mary Ann of similar appearance asking for an arsenic and soft-soap mixture to clean bedsteads and destroy bugs makes one suspicious. We know she did this towards the end of May, 1872, some six weeks before Charles Edward's death, and we know she had some of the mixture earlier, just after the series of three deaths which ended with that of Joseph Nattrass on Easter Monday, 1st April, 1872. But using the lethal mixture for this purpose could well have been reasonably common, and certainly in the north-east the christian names, Mary Ann, were popular choices. When Mary Ann was eighteen and living in Murton Colliery there was a girl in a house next door and in one next to it with exactly the same name, Mary Ann Robson.

The next poisoning after January, 1869, which we know of and for which she could have been responsible, was that of her friend Margaret Cotton at North Walbottle in March, 1870, and the arsenic for this could have come from the doctor's surgery in Spennymoor where Mary Ann was working about this time. The buyer in the Newcastle shop wanted only the arsenic mixture and wanted it then and there, so if it were Mary Ann she could have got it with Robinson and his two remaining children in mind, if he would agree to everyone being insured, but he would not. Early 1869 was the time when she was running into money difficulties in the Robinson household and beginning to tamper with payment entries.

For what it is worth, and it could be conclusive, a week or so after the hearing an Elizabeth Robson in Newcastle affirmed that she was the witness and that the purchaser had not been Mary Ann Cotton. The prosecution did not call Detchon at the trial for the murder of Charles Edward when, of course, they could prove that arsenic had been bought locally only some six weeks before death. Detchon upset Mary Ann. She expected him at the trial and she was concerned enough to alter her hair style. Again, this could be as much to try to show him he was wrong as to mislead him that she was not the woman he remembered.

The thrice-given evidence of Jane Hedley that Mary Ann had arsenic mixture left after the three poisonings was never followed up, although obviously the prosecution could not offer any evidence of purchase prior to these deaths, other than the possible one in Newcastle in January, 1869.

Clearly Kilburn and Chalmers never gave murder a thought. Chalmers, even though puzzled by the lack of effect of the medicine given to young Frederick Cotton, readily accepted the sudden fatal change in the condition of the baby less than three weeks later. He had no doubt but that the child died of teething convulsions. Mary Ann herself seems to have been worried about the reaction of others to the sudden change. She did not want Mary Tate to bring anyone in to see the child. The women neighbours were shocked, however, and this could have been material for Riley to ponder later on.

Mary Ann was a lone person, a secret person, no matter how neighbours milled around. The fact that they did so shows she had either a friendly side or qualities which they admired or which drew them to her. One gets the impression that she had a strong personality; most of the neighbours seem to have done her bidding. Her nursing experience would gain her some respect, and perhaps hints and partial disclosures of past husbands and different places would intrigue the women. Her sexuality could have been attractive. But no one penetrated, or was admitted to, her deep motivating thoughts. There was no confidante. She could hold her tongue. Surrounded by trust, she decided and acted furtively.

She must have been administering arsenic to her baby and to her recent lover Joe Nattrass at the same time, with Mary Tate sometimes in the house. The last drink given to the child would be after both doctors had been and Sarah Smith and Mary Tate had left and she was on her own. The fit she had could have been a cracking under the strain of a deed almost accomplished with so many people about, or just a further, almost intuitive act, both distracting and sympathy-gaining, in her long lone part. In this case, though, the too-sudden deterioration alarmed her and made her apprehensive of the doctor.

Mary Ann was now finished with the Auckland district, after only a year or so in it. She left it for good that evening. She had travelled around far more than most people in like social circumstances, and it ended with a miserable journey back to the county gaol through darkness, cold and snow. There were crowds to see her leave Bishop Auckland with her baby, and people were waiting at Durham station to see her arrive there.

There were many tales about her now, tales which were long to outlive the amply reported evidence. Even today there are people who believe that Mary Ann Cotton lured children to their deaths by her beguiling appearance and words and by giving little rewards for going messages for her, or that she ran a baby-farm taking in unwanted children for twenty pounds or so and disposing of them so cleverly that charges could not be brought against her. One lady in Bowburn, County Durham, told me that Mary Ann was the cause of her father being teetotal for life. When he was a boy Mary Ann had asked him to go for some beer for her and given him a sup which made him unforgettably ill.

That last day in Bishop Auckland there were rumours that the formidable Charles Russell, Q.C., would lead for the Treasury at the assizes and that the case to be heard first would be that of the last death, that of seven-year-old Charles Edward Cotton.

Running parallel with the horror at what Mary Ann seemed to have done was a disbelief that such actions were possible, and a growing sympathy for her because of her lone, defenceless position. Some gentlemen and tradesmen in Bishop Auckland formed a committee to raise funds for her defence. They advertised in newspapers saying John Leng of the Sun Inn would receive donations. They retained a local solicitor and had hopes of employing Thomas Campbell Foster of the northern circuit to defend 'this unhappy woman'. There was little time – only a week – before she appeared at the spring assizes on 5th March.

At Durham General Sessions, prior to the assizes, a thirty-year-old married woman was given seven years' penal servitude for taking four pairs of trousers which were hanging in a shop-doorway in Gateshead. There were seven years of penal servitude also for a sailor who broke into a shop in South Shields and stole twenty-nine shillings; for a forty-seven-year-old spinster who stole a pair of boots in Sunderland, and for a thirty-four-year-old widow who stole a purse, twenty-three shillings and a handkerchief in Bishop Auckland. Three magistrates, two of them clergymen, sentenced a forty-two-year-old labourer to twelve months' hard labour for taking some bones away from Monkwearmouth station in Sunderland.

Before she came to West Auckland Mary Ann had avoided the frightening law by moving around; by enough knowledge of arsenic and fever to deceive doctors; by the cover given by insanitary conditions and the mortality rate; and by the innocence and trust of others. However, in contradistinction to the severity of punishment for stealing, there was a revulsion against sentencing a woman to be hanged. There was Christian concern over judicial killing, and impressive urging to have such killing brought to an end could be read in the press. Twenty-two years earlier, at an inquest held on a farmer of Kelloe, in County Durham, who died from arsenic poisoning, the jury returned a verdict of wilful murder against his wife. At the assizes the grand jury threw out the bill against her. The last execution of a woman at Durham had been that of Mary Nicholson, as long ago as 1799, for the poisoning of her mistress. The case was referred to twelve judges and she was not sentenced for a year. Her execution was not expeditious, either.

But before we hear of the rhetoric and ingenuities at Mary Ann Cotton's trial at the spring assizes of 1873, and of what followed, perhaps we should look, as well as we can, at her life before she went to West Auckland.

CHAPTER FOUR

The story before West Auckland

Mary Ann Cotton would think of herself for most of the time as Mary Ann Robson or Mary Ann Mowbray. She was born in 1832, almost certainly late in October, in the small pit village of Low Moorsley, then in the parish of Houghton-le-Spring in County Durham. Pits in the area had been in operation for some twenty years. There were only four or five streets in the village, directly and simply named Low Row, High Row, Back Row, Front Row. In spite of its name, Low Moorsley is on highish ground, below High Moorsley. The land falls away to the east, to Hetton-le-Hole. To the north and north-east there is an open view from the village over good arable country to East Rainton and down to Houghton-le-Spring.

On 11th November Mary Ann was baptized at Rainton Chapel, now St Mary's Church, West Rainton. Her parents, Michael and Margaret Robson, were very young: it could be that her father was only seventeen when she was baptized. His description is the same as most in the register: pitman. In the 1841 census the parents' ages were entered as twenty-five and Mary Ann's as eight. But in the 1851 census her mother's age jumps thirteen years to thirty-eight; in the 1861 census forty-seven was given as her age: so it looks as if her mother could well have been the older parent.

Shortly after Mary Ann's birth the Robsons moved to East Rainton, a little over a mile away. Michael Robson worked at the Hazard pit, one of three local pits. Margaret Robson had been born at Tanfield, between Stanley and Gateshead, but her father, called Lonsdale, had worked at the Hazard pit as a brakesman for many years. It has been said that Michael Robson worked on the Hazard shafts as a sinker, but the description he gave when his next two children were baptized was again pitman. A sinker usually gave his specific description.

The second daughter, given the same name as her mother,

was born on 28th July, 1834, and Mary Ann's brother, Robert, on 5th October, 1835. If the entry in the 1841 census was the correct one, the young Mrs Robson had three children by the time she was twenty. It is pretty certain she had no more. Only Mary Ann and Robert were registered in the 1841 census, and as, later, Mary Ann, looking back, referred only to her beloved brother, it seems probable that little Margaret did not live long.

East Rainton, a pleasant village today, lies midway between Sunderland and Durham city. It had a population of some fifteen hundred in those days, nearly all pitfolk. The Robsons probably lived in a cottage at the Durham end of the village, near to the old church school and on the site of the present school. Pontop pit was not far away and it is thought the cottage itself was called Pontop. It was two-roomed and there was a garden between it and the church school. Sanitation was a hole in the ground with a portable hut over it. When the hole had to be filled in another was dug and the hut moved over it. A cottage outside the village, on the corner of Quarry House Lane and the Hetton road, is also mentioned as the Robsons' home. The remains of the old Hazard pit, not all overgrown – the pit was worked for over a hundred years – are a few hundred yards away from this site.

The Wesleyans, as was usual in colliery villages, were the first to provide a place of worship in East Rainton. Two old cottages in the centre of the village were transformed into a chapel, rebuilt in 1889. Michael Robson is said to have taken a class at the chapel, and even conducted the choir. Mary Ann, quite definitely, was to take a Sunday-school class when in her teens.

I think one can state she was a strikingly pretty child. An old inhabitant, spoken to in the 1920s, remembered her fine dark eyes and said her exceptional prettiness was talked about.

The Robsons were living at Murton early in 1841 when Mary Ann was eight, and I fancy they had not been there long. There is a tradition of Mary Ann living at East Rainton. It is usually given that she was born there, although Murton occasionally gets the award – the first police report on Mary Ann said she was born at Murton. Until I eventually arrived at the West Rainton church baptism register Low Moorsley had remained unsullied, not even suspected as the birthplace.

East Rainton is also one of the places where she is supposed to have sent a boy friend to his death by pushing him down a pitshaft. The belief that she did such a deed persists. At East Rainton it is thought it was either at the Hazard or the Dun Well pit. At South Hetton, two to three miles away, I have been told the shaft was that of the Hetton Lyons pit.

So by 1841 Michael Robson, probably twenty-five years old, was working at Murton – suddenly a place of enginemen, firemen and, most of all, pit-sinkers. Michael was one of these.

The collieries in the East Rainton area were in the North Hetton group, their shafts sunk through limestone. There had been fears that coal beneath the magnesium limestone would be of poor quality, but it was found that this wasn't so and that the coal was plentiful. The coal seams ran deeper underground to the east towards the coast and this increased the difficulties of shaft-sinking. After the South Hetton shaft was sunk successfully in 1831, thoughts turned a further two miles east, to near the old farming hamlet of Murton, where the coal was some hundreds of feet below water-bearing strata and sand. The sinking of a pitshaft there was expected to be a formidable undertaking: it proved to be worse than the surveyors and engineers had feared. From the start in 1838 it took five years to reach the coal: twice water exploded deep in the shafts. It was many more years before coal was being won regularly at Murton, and it was many more still before there was another sinking through limestone.

The workings and the community were known as Murton New Winning up to mid-1845. In 1841 there were 500 people living there, a five-fold increase on the old farming population. Because of the enormous cost of opening the pit – five times that of others in the area – the idea of continuous coal-winning was conceived and put into operation early in the 1850s. The coal was drawn out twenty-four hours a day, too, except when men were being lowered or raised. But long before that the traditional price of coal had been paid by the Robson family, and one can only guess at the effect of that on the character of Mary Ann.

The Robsons lived in Durham Place, one of the first of the new streets to be built. They were terrace houses, of course, double-storeyed, of rough stone: they were demolished in the early 1950s. The Robsons' house was probably a corner one, number 25, between the present Welfare Hall and the Travellers' Rest public house. In the early days of the colliery, the Travellers' Rest had a company shop. Mary Ann went to school at Murton and to the Wesleyan Sunday school.

Michael Robson was killed early in 1842. He slipped and fell down a shaft when repairing a pulley wheel. His age on the death certificate is thirty, not twenty-six which would have agreed with the census of the year before.

Margaret Robson did not remain a widow long. Her second husband, George Stott, a Gateshead man, said later he had brought up Mary Ann from being a child. He, too, was a miner at Murton and a Methodist. He was younger than Margaret, five years by the 1851 census, three years by the 1861.

In 1844 Murton men joined the great strike. New men were brought in and there were many evictions. I have not seen any indication that Mary Ann's family was turned out.

When she was sixteen or so Mary Ann got a position as nursemaid to the family of Edward Potter in South Hetton. Potter was colliery manager and a very important man in the area. He had been in charge of the shaft-sinking operations at Murton. He lived at South Hetton House, within the pit-top compound. Known locally as 'the Hall', this house is on the east side of Front Street, South Hetton's main street. Margaret Potter had been bearing a child a year for some years; the eldest would be twelve when Mary Ann came to the house.

She was there for two to three years. Mrs Potter has been quoted speaking of the girl's beauty and saying that a curate fell in love with her. A Wesleyan Sunday school had been started in the village in 1845 and Mary Ann became a teacher there. She was to look back on these pre-marriage days in Murton and South Hetton as happy and untroubled.

After leaving South Hetton House Mary Ann began to learn to be a dressmaker. About this time her mother was attempting to run a small school. Mary Ann's brother, Robert Robson, is entered in the 1851 census return: his age, fifteen; description, coal-miner. Mary Ann was eighteen then.

Now William Mowbray comes on the scene. He was a labourer, one of the many men drawn to the new working at Murton. The accounts in the press in 1872 and 1873 of Mary Ann's life state that he was from Peterborough, but in the 1861 census Shotley in Northumberland is given as his birthplace. His father was a cartwright.

He married Mary Ann on 18th July, 1852. He gave his age as twenty-six, an age confirmed by the 1861 census in which he is entered as thirty-five. On his death early in 1865, not quite four years later, his age was given as forty-seven. It could well be that Mary Ann wanted then to make it appear he was older than he was.

I get the impression that Mowbray did his best in those times, and that his moving from job to job and place to place was not because he could not hold down a job but because he was trying to improve things. I also fancy that he had made Mary Ann pregnant before they were married and that she married in disgrace.

The information gained when police and reporters were probing into her past was that the marriage took place at St Andrew's Church in Gallowgate, Newcastle, the church in which she bigamously married Frederick Cotton eighteen years later in 1870. In fact, they were married in Newcastle Register Office. Each gave the address of Westgate, Newcastle. Mary Ann said she was twenty-one.

Mowbray, of course, could have been a non-believer and stood out for a register office marriage, but it is more likely that Mary Ann was going to have a child, and that to chapel-going people a church wedding would have seemed sacrilegious. For many, many years, certainly in my lifetime, a register office marriage in the north-east was looked upon by many as a prosaic, joyless substitute for the real thing, the resort of those who had to get married.

And the choosing of the privacy of the big city of Newcastle, some twenty miles to the north, rather than the small community in which she lived; her giving of the independent age of twenty-one when she was nineteen, and the going far away after the marriage, indicates family dismay and dissension. It is possible that Mary Ann's feeling of exclusion began at this time. Perhaps there would have been some forbearance if Michael Robson had not been killed.

Mowbray and Mary Ann broke completely with the north-east, going to the west country. There, in Somerset and Cornwall, Mowbray got work with contracting firms, probably navvying at first. He became timekeeper for a railway-construction firm, and they were settled for some time in Penzance. Mowbray could well have heard about that part of the country from the Cornishmen working at Murton. Teams of Cornishmen moved to the north-east as experts in shaft-sinking, and tin-miners had been lured to Murton to help break the 1844 strike.

So Mary Ann had her first children away from her mother and old friends. After some years her mother did visit her, staying three months in Penzance. Then when Mrs Stott returned to Murton Mary Ann and Mowbray followed within a few weeks. They had been away for more than four years. She returned with one child, called Mary Ann, and she said she had had four others – some accounts say a more likely three others and all had died. These deaths are sometimes included in the tally of those poisoned, but there is no evidence of any sort to support this.

On 5th April, 1857, the Mowbrays' first child to be born in the north-east, Margaret Jane, was baptized at St Andrew's church, Dalton-le-Dale, then the parish church for Murton. Mowbray was now a storekeeper at the colliery. This St Andrew's church was the obvious one for the Mowbrays to have been married in, but there is no entry in the register. It seems that little Margaret Jane too, like her sisters born in the south-west, had a short life. She was not living at the time of the 1861 census, and Mary Ann was to give the same christian names to another daughter born to her in the autumn of 1861.

By September, 1858, the Mowbrays must have made the short move to South Hetton, as on the 26th of that month their daughter Isabella was born there. She was baptized at the Holy Trinity church, then the chapelry of South Hetton in Easington parish, a week before Christmas. Mowbray was then described as a stoker. Isabella lived longer with Mary Ann than any child – she reached the age of nine.

On 24th June, 1860, the child Mary Ann had brought with her from Penzance, Mary Ann, was buried at the South Hetton church. The colliery doctor, Samuel Broadbent, certified that gastric fever was the cause of the four-year-old girl's death.

In the 1861 census return the Mowbrays are shown as living in a public-house in South Hetton, with Mary Ann's mother and step-father next door. In the village it is thought that the public house was the Screeners' Arms, but this is not mentioned in directories of the period, although later, in the 1870s, there was a Screenmen's Arms in Gale Street, just off Front Street, property which is now pulled down. The Wesleyan Methodist chapel in Front Street was very near to the Mowbrays' public house: the pubs adjacent to the chapel in the maps of the period were the Hope and Anchor and the Butchers' Arms. George Stott was certainly landlord of the Butchers' Arms a few years later. This pub was at the junction of Front Street and Clarence Street. Stott also kept, at other times, the Bird Inn and the Bradyll Arms.

On 1st October, 1861, the second Margaret Jane was born.

Mowbray's description at the baptism two months later was fireman; and it was stoker when Mary Ann's first known boy, John Robert, born 22nd November, 1863, was baptized, again at the Holy Trinity chapelry.

Certainly in this period Mowbray left his colliery work at South Hetton and went to sea as a stoker on the screw steamer, *Newburn*, trading from Sunderland. The master was an uncle of Mary Ann's, John Hulbard, married to her mother's sister. It looks as if Mowbray was going to sea when his home was at South Hetton, but after the birth of the boy the Mowbrays left the colliery community and moved to Sunderland.

The boy died within the year. His body was brought to South Hetton and was buried in the Holy Trinity churchyard on 22nd September, 1864. The register gives his home as Bishopwearmouth, the part of Sunderland on the south side of the Wear.

Then in January, 1865, Mowbray himself died. He had been home with an injured foot when he was stricken by an attack of diarrhoea so violent that he died within a few hours. On 18th January his body too, was brought to South Hetton. In the burial register his abode was given as Hendon, Sunderland, and his age as forty-seven. Mary Ann would be thirty-two at the time.

A Dr Gammage certified the deaths as due to gastric fever and diarrhoea. Diarrhoea was often stated to be a cause of death then: it was generally spread by flies infecting exposed food, and it became less frequent as middens were cleared away. It is, too, a symptom of arsenic poisoning.

Mary Ann is said to have taken the deaths badly, especially that of her husband to whom she had been married for more than twelve years. Thornton Hall, writing in 1931 a series of articles about the poisonings, said that when Mowbray looked to be dying Dr Gammage himself was affected by Mary Ann's distress. Shortly after Mowbray's death the doctor heard singing as he passed Mary Ann's house and, peering through the drawn blinds, he saw the new widow pirouetting before a mirror as she sang a popular song. It is a possible picture, although Hall settles quickly for a few facts and lets invention rip.

It seems probable that Mary Ann's standard of living worsened in Sunderland. For the first time Mowbray was not in regular work; his health was deteriorating, and there would not be long-known neighbours to help. Then there were three children, two of them young enough to keep his wife at home.

If Mowbray died there was the large amount of £35 insurance money to be received from the British Prudential. It looks suspicious. But where had she picked up her knowledge of arsenic? Had it been used medicinally when she was at the Potters?' Could it be that when she was in Devon and Cornwall she was near to mineral deposits of the stuff and learnt something about it?

Mary Ann left Sunderland for a time when Mowbray died. With the two children she went to Seaham Harbour, a coal-port some five miles down the coast from Hendon. She took a room there with a view of the sea, almost overlooking the harbour – a front room on the ground floor of property known as Bolton's Houses in North Terrace. Other tenements stretched to the infirmary at the corner. The two-storeyed building, which is still there, was next door to the Lord Seaham Inn, facing Terrace Green and the cliff tops.

It was here she met Joseph Nattrass who was staying at Bolton's with his brother. Nattrass, from Ryhope, between Sunderland and Seaham, would be twenty-eight at the time, and he was engaged to a local girl, Mary Thubron. It seems that Mary Ann fell in love with him and that there was an affair, but this did not stop his marriage, and after it he moved away to work at Shildon colliery, near to Bishop Auckland.

One must wonder if the affair had its effect on the two children: it could well, of course, have had nothing to do with what happened to them. The younger child, the second Margaret Jane, aged three and a half, died of gastric fever after being ill for two or three days. She was attended by a Seaham doctor, and Dr Gammage, on a visit from Sunderland, was also called in by Mary Ann. Margaret Jane was buried at South Hetton on 2nd May, 1865. And the other child, six-year-old Isabella, the surviving child of the eight or nine born to Mary Ann, was taken by her grandmother, Mrs Stott, then living at New Seaham. So Mary Ann was on her own for the first time in her life. It is thought that at Seaham she made an attempt to earn a living by dressmaking, but I wonder about that old infirmary at the end of North Terrace. When she returned to Sunderland she was to work well in the old infirmary there.

The Sunderland Infirmary, House of Recovery for the Cure of Contagious Fever, Dispensary and Humane Society – in recent times St Mary's Catholic School – was at the foot of old Chester Road. Mary Ann worked in the House of Recovery, the Fever House, which had twenty beds. Patients paid one-and-sixpence a day; the parish paid for paupers. Bedsheets were changed once a fortnight, and patients' linen every four days. There were no baths, and, when possible, patients were taken in cabs to the public baths. A nurse was paid a shilling a day, plus board and lodging when on duty. She had to wash out her ward by seven in the morning during the summer, and by eight in the winter, and serve breakfast within the next hour. Beverages, even for children, were beer, beer gruel, barley gruel and water. There was no small isolation ward. There was a small room upstairs for operations. Medicines were left in this room for the nurses to collect, at any time of day or night.

Until shortly before Mary Ann was employed there, the Fever House had been separate from the infirmary and dispensary, being entered by its own outside door. But such was the prevalence of fever that the risk of breaking a way between the two was taken and for a time an infirmary ward was taken over. In spite of an outbreak of typhoid fever in the infirmary the number of deaths there in 1865 was exceptionally low; the rate of 3.7 per cent was the lowest since the building was put up in 1823. Among fever patients the mortality rate was the highest, 22.4 per cent. The report for 1865 says this great number of deaths was due to overcrowding and to patients being received when they were beyond aid. All the nurses but one caught typhoid fever that year. Mary Ann, it seems, worked well and bravely. Later, the doctor in charge praised her, saying she was one of the best nurses.

At the assizes a witness said Mary Ann worked at the old infirmary for nearly a year, but the period between the death of Margaret Jane at Seaham and her second marriage was less than four months. Of course she may have worked on for a time after her re-marriage. She was certainly there long enough to impress the doctors.

She had seen quite a lot of suffering and dying by now, but she must have appeared to be sympathetic. There are many references to her concern for those she tended. One of the fever patients who was impressed was George Ward, an engineer and a single man of her own age, thirty-two – a well-built and normally strong man. On his discharge they were married at St Peter's church, Monkwearmouth, on the north side of the Wear at Sunderland. That was on 28th August, 1865. It was the first of Mary Ann's three marriages in fine old churches. St

Peter's, indeed, had been there since the seventh century. Bede, the historian, lived there when a boy in its earliest days. Dame Dorothy Street, nearby the church, was given as the address of each, but Ward took her to live on the south side in the heart of old Sunderland, in Ettrick Place at the top of Grey Street, between High Street East and Coronation Street.

Eighteen sixty-five was an eventful year for Mary Ann, and the marriage was not the end. The union cannot have been a happy one. Ward was either unable to get work, or not strong enough to work after the fever, and Mary Ann found herself again impoverished in Sunderland. And after bearing so many children by Mowbray, she had none by Ward. Perhaps he was a disappointment sexually. If she resented having to look after children here was a time alone with a new man, but something was wrong for her.

By November Ward was receiving 4s. a week parish relief and late in the month he was seen by Dr Dixon, soon to be house surgeon at the infirmary. In mid-December a second doctor, Maling, house surgeon when Ward was in the fever hospital, also saw him. He got this special attention because of Maling wanting to help one of his old nurses.

Ward, 'well proportioned and muscular', complained of nose-bleedings and 'want of strength'. The doctors were puzzled, Dixon especially. He saw Ward on three successive days and after an examination of lungs, heart and liver, and persistent questioning, all of which seems to have disturbed Mary Ann, Dixon felt satisfied at finding that there was enlargement and congestion of the liver. He asked Mary Ann to apply twelve leeches. She assured him she could do this all right. He told her to send for him at the infirmary should anything go wrong. The following day Dixon sent his assistant, a Mr Coul, who found that the leech bites had bled rather freely during the night and he put on a fresh dressing. The next morning Dixon called and, to his own great annoyance and Mary Ann's embarrassment, found Maling attending to Ward who was weak from loss of blood. Dixon was out of temper with her and she explained that she had no one to send for him, that she couldn't leave her husband, and that a neighbour, who had called in accidentally, had gone for Dr Maling on her own. Dixon continued to attend Ward until he was able to sit up at the fire, and then, because of Mary Ann's obvious preference for Maling, he withdrew. Later, Maling too, withdrew: before he did so he was aware that there were symptoms of paralysis.

The unfortunate and perplexed Ward was unwell for months. In May, 1866, feeling a little better but frustrated and bitter, he complained about Dixon to the relieving officer, a Mr Humphrey, saying that the doctor's inattention at the time of the leech-bites was responsible for his lingering illness and the paralysis of his hands and feet. He said Dixon had been sent for more than once at the time and hadn't come, and that Maling, who had sewn up the leech-holes, had told him that if he hadn't been attended to he would have died. Mary Ann joined in the denunciation of Dixon. Perhaps she had to, as Ward obviously thought she had sent for Dixon. One imagines she expected that the complaint would stop at Humphrey, after helping to ensure that they continued to receive the four shillings a week. But the relieving officer reported the complaint to the Sunderland board of guardians, and appeared before them at their next meeting. The matter was reported in the local press under the heading: 'A Statement Against a Medical Man'. Some members of the board regretted the public slur on Dixon's reputation when they were hearing only Ward's account. The infirmary committee was asked to investigate, and Dixon made a longish statement, called, 'Facts in the Case of George Ward'. A fortnight after hearing of Ward's complaint the guardians agreed it was entirely disproved and Dixon was cleared of any charge against him.

Dixon could have been near to preventing a number of murders: of the various doctors in Mary Ann's life he was the least satisfied with appearances. As it was, his probing, in the end, got him a bad public name for a time. I wonder what he thought about it all six years later when news was breaking about Mary Ann! It has been said that both he and Maling then declared that arsenical poisoning would have accounted for the symptoms. In evidence to the infirmary committee Maling had said he did not think the paralysis could have come from the leech bites.

But poor George Ward was a worse victim. The immediate acceptance of Dixon's statement meant loss of sympathy. Did he turn on Mary Ann asking why she had not sent for Dixon, why she had said she had, or allowed him to believe she had? Perhaps he just accepted that Dixon had to make such a statement to get in the clear. Ward lived on for five months or so after his complaint. He was buried on 21st October, 1866, in

Sunderland cemetery, then known as Sunderland-by-the-Sea cemetery, to the south of the town in Grangetown. The word 'fever', is pencilled by his name in the cemetery register. Five cholera victims are entered on the same page. Ward was thirty-three. He could have had no idea of the final dismal year of living he was entering when his hopeful eyes and thoughts began to linger on the nurse.

Mary Ann was known to attend regularly for a time at Sans Street Mission Hall, the mother chapel of Wesleyan Methodists in the town. She could have begun to worship there when she was married to Ward, as the hall was near to where they lived. This Mission seated nearly 2,500 people and was a popular meeting-place for many years. It is now twin cinemas.

She moved out of the house in Ettrick Place after Ward's death to one nearby, in Sussex Street at its junction with Borough Road, next door to Humphrey, the relieving officer. As she can have been there for only two months or so after Ward died she might have lived in it before, when she was a nurse, and it could, indeed, have been her Hendon home with Mowbray.

St Thomas's Church Institute and St Thomas's National School were in Sussex Street and by the time Mary Ann had reached West Auckland the house, No. 9, was the residence of a curate of the church. In 1893 Canon Arthur Nesham Bax in his first curacy was sent by his vicar to live in this house, which had two upper floors and a basement and was in a rough and poor area. It had a bad reputation because of Mary Ann. From time to time a prematurely old woman who helped to look after him would come and announce that she had just seen Mary Ann Cotton leading a child across the yard.

At the end of November, 1866, twenty-seven-year-old Hannah Robinson died in the up-river Sunderland suburb of Pallion leaving her husband, James, and five children. Robinson, a shipwright at a small yard on the Wear at Pallion, almost immediately advertised for a housekeeper. Mary Ann applied, got the position and moved into the household well before Christmas. She entered, a forerunner of death for some of the children left by the young wife, and one who, at the same time, beguiled the father.

The first child to die was the baby, John Robinson, ten months old. He was buried at Bishopwearmouth cemetery on 23rd December, three weeks after his mother. A week after Mary Ann's arrival he was taken ill and twenty hours after the first sign of illness he was dead, after a succession of convulsions. He died during the night and the doctor, Dr Shaw, of Ayres Quay, Deptford, who had been sent for, arrived too late. He certified gastric fever as the cause of death.

Mary Ann was pregnant by Robinson by early March. About this time she was called away to look after her mother at New Seaham. Nine days later Mrs Stott died – this was on 15th March, 1867. Her age has been given as fifty-four which is in accord with the return in the 1851 census. Mrs Stott's death was a surprise one, and as Mary Ann had said to unbelieving neighbours that she feared her mother was going to die and there seemed no likelihood of this at the time, this death, too, is regarded as a possible poisoning. The neighbours, too, resented Mary Ann's seizing of some clothing and bed linen. And Mary Ann annoyed her stepfather, although there does not seem to have been much sympathy between them at any time. He is quoted as saying that he did not want her in the house again.

There is no mention of Mary Ann receiving any insurance money on her mother's death, or of any rift between them. The mother could have been outspoken and less considerate in her remarks about the succession of deaths. Perhaps she was bedridden or in need of a long rest, and Mary Ann could have been wanting to get back to Robinson quickly to establish further her position there. Her life in that household was the best, materially, she had had or was to have with men. But her references to her mother imply feeling, trust, and a deprivation when her mother died. In a letter from prison she wrote: 'You speak of mother, had i my mother i should not been hear . . . but thanke god she is i hope in heaven, she left evry resons to beleav she was happy.'

Mrs Stott's death meant the death sentence for Isabella Mowbray, then nine. Mary Ann took her back with her to Pallion, where, like the Robinson children, Isabella was now without female protection and love.

In April two more of the children were taken ill – James, who was six, and eight-year-old Elizabeth. There was nothing sudden about the development of their sickness: Dr Shaw, some days, called twice to see them. Mary Ann prepared the neighbours for Isabella going down with the same sickness, and this the girl duly did. She was ill before the little boy died. He was buried on 21st April, Elizabeth on 26th April, and Isabella on 2nd May, all in Bishopwearmouth cemetery. All had similar symptoms: rolling about in bed, foaming at the mouth and retching, especially after being given a drink. Gastric fever was given as the cause of the deaths. Superintendent Henderson, in his report to the Home Office in 1872, showed that he was next to certain that the three children had been poisoned. He wanted their bodies exhumed.

Mary Ann played her part well, retaining the affection, confidence and support of Robinson. It seemed as if she was going to catch the fever herself and Robinson wanted to send for Shaw again, but Mary Ann would not let him do this and she recovered. She was in a highly emotional state at the time of the deaths and funerals: spells of depression and of hurrying about followed each other. She was critical of her behaviour and said she should have done better, and Robinson had to talk her out of doing injury to herself. Robinson, too, defended her against the declared mistrust of his three sisters – defended her angrily. These women seem to have been the first to feel fairly strongly that Mary Ann was a poisoner.

Robinson, a hard-working, careful man needed a woman partner. He had money in the post office savings bank and he was buying his house through a building society. All the same, his marriage to Mary Ann was late in the day: opposition from his sisters could well have caused delay, and it seems they did not know of the wedding until afterwards. Mary Ann was five months pregnant when they married. The ceremony was at Bishopwearmouth Church, near to the old infirmary, on 11th August, 1867. It could well be significant that the deaths of the three children followed her knowledge that she was pregnant to Robinson and so almost certain to marry him. They were both thirty-four years old, and they gave separate addresses, nearer to the church, 21, Sans Street for Robinson, and High Street West for Mary Ann. Robinson signed his hand well and plainly. She gave her name as Mowbray, which she was to do again when she married Cotton three years later. Probably she did not tell Robinson about Ward.

Their child, another girl, was born on 29th November. Mary Ann used a small number of girls' names and on 18th February the baby was baptised Mary Isabella at St Andrew's Church in the shipyard district of Deptford on the town side of Pallion. Mary Ann again gave her maiden name as Mowbray. The baby died a few days later another victim of gastric fever and was buried on 1st March. There is a name disparity in the burial register: Margaret instead of Mary. The child was the fifth and last to die when Mary Ann was living with Robinson. He said later, that, at the time, he would not let his mind dwell on some thoughts: that he dare not. Two of Robinson's children escaped, as well as Robinson himself, and a second child she had to him.

She had suggested soon after joining the household that the children should be insured but he would not do this, although it appears that he received payments from some society on their deaths and that he passed this over to Mary Ann, who also received insurance money for Isabella. Robinson also refused to have himself insured. She eventually tried to insure him herself without his knowing, but he found out and stopped her.

At some time during her life with Robinson, almost certainly in 1868 after the death of the baby, she had a spell of employment at Sunderland's new Royal Infirmary in Durham Road.

Early in 1869 one of the two Sunderland building societies the Robinsons were in, Mr Trewhitt's, in making up the pass book found that amounts paid had been made greater by the addition of ten-shilling strokes. Robinson was again quick to defend his wife: he maintained that the amounts in the book had been paid in by her and that the society was mistaken. The matter angered him so much that he told Mary Ann to withhold further payments. In October, however, he became apprehensive when the society threatened some action and said to his wife she had better let them have the payments now – they totalled £5. He received the first real shaking of his confidence in Mary Ann when she informed him that the society did not want the accumulated payments until the following week. A few days later he found she had been trying to borrow £5 from a loan office, giving the names of his brother-in-law and uncle as guarantors. Then, questioned, his son told him that his stepmother had been sending him to the pawnbrokers.

Robinson's whole edifice of trust and confidence collapsed. He said that he and Mary Ann would have to separate. She promised to get the £5 from her stepfather, but Robinson was finished. He insisted that she did some explaining to someone in Sunderland and he arranged to meet her after he had finished work on Deptford Bridge. She was not there, and on going home he found she had left, taking her surviving child by him. He soon learnt that there were debts, that he was £7 in arrears at the other building society (Mr Wayman's), and that in spite of the amount entered in his post office savings book there was in fact next to nothing left in the account. Robinson shut up the house and moved in with his married sister in Coronation Street, Sunderland. Later he set up home in Rosannah Street, Deptford, near his work.

What on earth did Mary Ann need the extra money for? There is no apparent exceptional reason. There was no poverty with Robinson – there would be more money coming into the household than into many nearby. Perhaps he was too thrifty and careful and did not give her enough to run the house. There is not the slightest evidence that she spent more than a normal amount on drink, or that she drank much at all. She was always neatly dressed and could well have had a better wardrobe than many, but her dressmaking ability should have kept down that cost. She had one expense, however, unusual for a working class wife especially one from a mining area: she had the habit of paying others to do housework. She did this when living in West Auckland where her Front Street house was said to be 'beautiful and clean', and when she had less money than she had in Pallion. Perhaps looking after children and making clothes absorbed what patience she had, and she wanted to be tidy, to look attractive, to be admired and to enjoy love-making. Even so, it is doubtful if any help for which she paid took up all the extra money she came by when with Robinson. It could have been that she was simply a bad manager and always needed more money. That she sometimes asked neighbours to bring in things for her, and sent children on messages to corner shops and gave them rewards, indicates that she could have been a poor shopper. In West Auckland there were those who remembered Frederick Cotton observing that his first wife could make a penny go further than Mary Ann could a shilling.

Robinson gave Mary Ann a real chance to change. She lived longer with him than with anyone but Mowbray. She had a rough time when she left him. She had no possessions – she sold what she had in Sussex Street when she moved in with Robinson – and she returned to South Hetton for a while, although there was no maternal home there now for her and she did not see her step-father. Then, probably unusually contrite, she came back to Pallion to try to make it up with Robinson. She found the door locked and assumed that it was locked only against her. She was hurt and made bitter.

A factor which could have deepened her resentment was the situation of the house, 14, Grace Street, Low Pallion. It was one of the bottom houses of three rows of isolated shipyard terrace houses which ran steeply down to the yards at the upriver extremity of Sunderland. She would have to turn away – surely conscious of neighbours – and trudge back up the long bank and into town. The burial register entry for the baby, John Robinson, gives Gray Street as the address. It seems there was no Gray Street in Pallion, and the similarity in sound to Grace Street could explain the entry. There is remembrance of her living in Grace Street and of attending the chapel in Dove Street higher up the bank. What is not easily explained away is the entry of High Pallion, (no street given), for nine-year-old Isabella. Grace Street was in deepest Low Pallion. I doubt if the Robinson family moved at that time of grave illness and death, and I doubt if Mary Ann would allow ailing Isabella to be housed elsewhere, out of sight in someone else's care – although this is not impossible. There is no remembrance of Mary Ann living anywhere else in Pallion than in Grace Street.

Robinson never spoke to her again, although he thought he saw her in Sans Street Chapel one Sunday evening. She wanted him very much to visit her in prison, but he wouldn't. His sisters, on reading the early reports of the West Auckland poisonings, and not knowing, of course, that Mary Ann Cotton and Mary Ann Robinson, their sister-in-law, were the same person, said to him that this was the way his children went, and that, 'thy Mary Ann could have done that'.

The period of Mary Ann's life between Robinson and Cotton is nearly always described as one of loose living. Thornton Hall says she lived with a sailor and then stole his possessions when he went back to sea. There could have been some loose living, but there was not much time for it. By April, 1870 she had held two positions in Sunderland long enough to impress her employers; she was working for a doctor in Spennymoor, and she was pregnant – by Frederick Cotton, one assumes.

When she could not get back with Robinson she went to see Maling and asked for his help in obtaining a position. And, with the Ward case evidently no detraction, he, mentioned her work as a nurse for him, and recommended her successfully to Edward Backhouse, a retired banker, whose house, Ashburne, in its own parkland, was one of the finest in the town. It is now the Sunderland School of Art and Design in Backhouse Park. Maling described Mary Ann as an active, clever person. The description is interesting: it is not conventional but carefully chosen. When she was was at Ashburne she attended Sans Street Chapel each Sunday.

Backhouse was a dedicated Quaker and a man of consequence. A few years before, with other Quaker gentlemen, he had made a round of some infamous public houses in the town at about midnight. What he saw led to the withholding of many licences and to the closing-down of the most notorious places. He was to plead, sincerely and well, with the Home Secretary to spare Mary Ann's life. In the mid-sixties he established in Borough Road the Smyrna House Home for Fallen Women, often called the Sunderland Penitentiary Home, and Mary Ann worked there for a while, either before or after Ashburne, probably in charge of the laundry. Smyrna House was very near to her old home in Sussex Street. The staff of Smryna House too, were to plead for mercy to be shown to her.

At the end of 1869 an event took place which might have come from a Victorian ballad. With her baby Mary Ann called on a friend in Johnson Street, Sunderland. Later, saying she wanted to slip out and post a letter, she left the child with her friend and did not return. The friend took the child to Robinson on the turn of the year. He was out at a watch-night service and when he got back to his sister's home in the early hours of New Year's Day, 1870, the child was there. This baby, which Mary Ann asked in vain to see when in prison, was one of two of her twelve children to live on, (I am assuming), after her death. The other child was the one born in Durham gaol. If one surmised that the death of every child was accidental or from natural causes there would remain this incident of child-desertion to explain away.

There is no indication of why her two jobs in Sunderland did not last long. There is evidence that there was no antipathy towards her by her employers, as both, particularly Backhouse, pleaded publicly for her. Probably she was restless after being her own mistress, and we know she was unhappy about her life with Robinson coming to an end. Maybe details of her three marriages and the high number of deaths began to infiltrate. She decided to leave Sunderland after some six years there during which ten people close to her had died – two of them when she was temporarily in the Seaham area.

She was not long in finding a life which suited her. She was introduced to Frederick Cotton early in 1870 by his sister, Margaret, a domestic servant and old friend who had been in service with her, almost certainly at the Potters' in South Hetton when they were both in their teens. She was known to the Cotton family as Mary Ann Mowbray. This ill-fated family

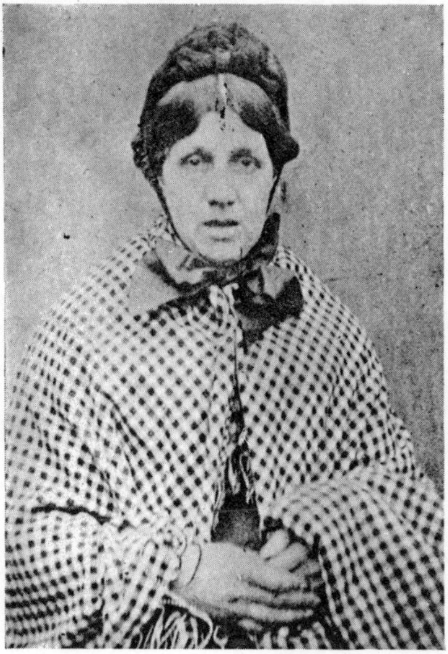

The actuality . . . taken by a Durham city photographer when Mary Ann was in custody in 1872 or 1873. She would be about forty years old.

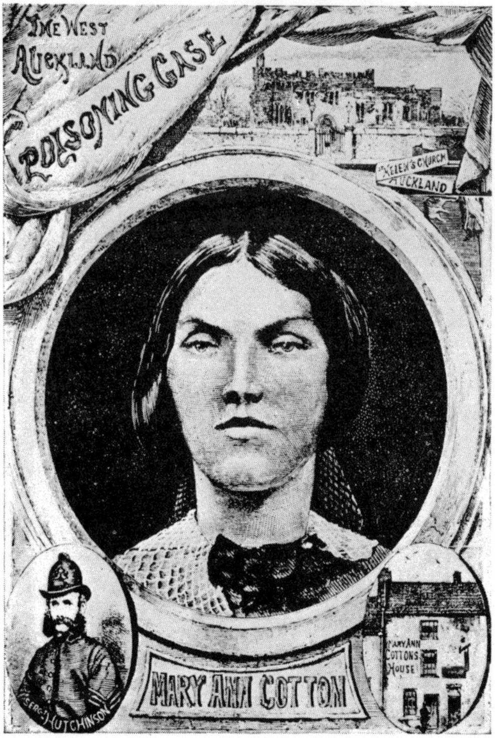

And the representation . . . The house was Mary Ann's last home, her second home in West Auckland. The boy, Charles Edward, died on the middle floor. The house is still lived in. The males of the unfortunate Cotton family and Joseph Nattrass were buried in St Helen's Auckland churchyard.

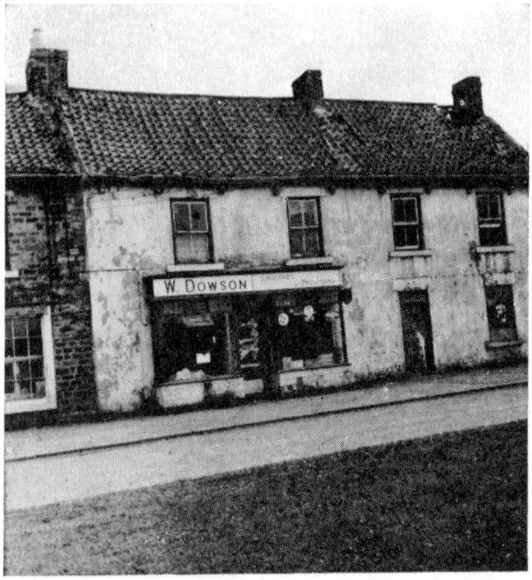

In 1872 this was Townend's chemist's shop by West Auckland green where Charles Edward was sent to buy the arsenic and soft soap.

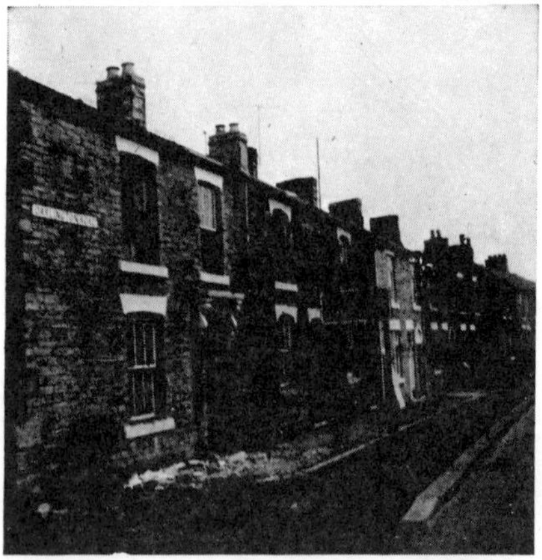

Darlington Road, West Auckland. The original name, Johnson Terrace, was on the square namestone near the roof.

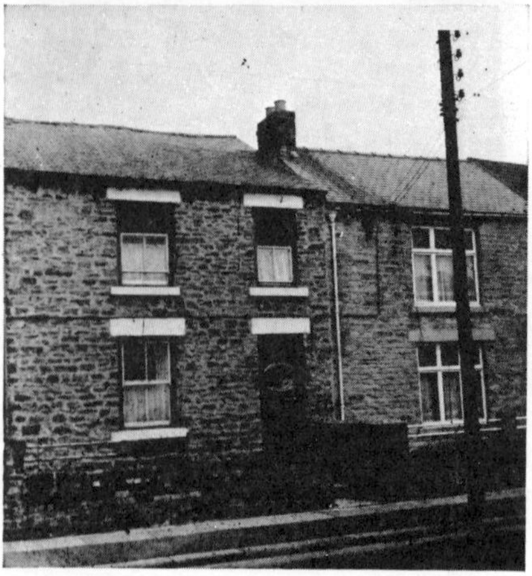

20, Johnson Terrace: Mary Ann Cotton's first home in West Auckland. Frederick Cotton, his eldest boy, Frederick, baby Robert, and Joseph Nattrass died here between September 1871 and April 1872.
(Pictures taken August 1972 just prior to demolition.)

lived at North Walbottle, a small isolated mining community in the Northumberland countryside, two miles north of the Tyne and six miles west of Newcastle. The village of Walbottle, on the course of Hadrian's Wall, was on lower ground a mile to the south, nearer the river. The North Walbottle community and their pit, the Coronation, were then and for many years known usually as the High Pit. The first deaths in the Cotton family were registered as taking place at High Pit, Walbottle.

Early in October, 1869, Frederick Cotton lived there with his thirty-four-year-old wife, Adelaide, and their four children – two girls and two boys. By March, 1872 all but one were dead, together with Cotton's sister Margaret and another child of Cotton's. The exception was the youngest of the four children, seven-year-old Charles Edward: his death, four months later, was to bring about Mary Ann's execution.

But Mary Ann had nothing to do with the early deaths: she was still in Sunderland when the eldest child, eleven-year-old Margaret, died of typhus fever on 9th October, and when Adelaide Cotton died of consumption on 19th December.

When Adelaide Cotton was dying Margaret left Stanhope Rectory in Weardale where she was laundry maid and came to look after things at Walbottle. Canon Clayton, Rector of Stanhope, said Margaret had about £60 in the bank, and that she had spoken to the other servants about Mary Ann. Frederick's brother Charles, writing from North Woolwich Road, Victoria Docks, London, to Hutchinson, the West Auckland police sergeant, said he felt Mary Ann had known his brother's family before the run of deaths at Walbottle, but known facts point to her knowing only Margaret then. Margaret had been employed at Stanhope Rectory since July 1866. Charles Cotton, then, in the autumn of 1872, was hitting out at Mary Ann by denying that she had approached him to take little Charles Edward or that there had ever been the slightest chance of his marrying her.

On 29th January, 1870, the remaining girl in the Cotton family, nine-year-old Adelaide Jane died, also of typhus fever. Mary Ann visited the household early in the year and could well have stayed for a while. On 25th March her friend, Margaret, died at the age of thirty-eight, after severe stomach pains. The cause of death was entered as pleuropneumonia. This death was so convenient for Mary Ann that one must be suspicious. She and Cotton were lovers by this time: by early April she was pregnant. I am assuming here, that Cotton was the father of the child, Robert Robson Cotton, born in January 1871.

But she did not move permanently into the household after the death of Margaret; in fact she moved a good distance away, to Spennymoor, some twenty miles south, between Durham city and Bishop Auckland where she was employed as housekeeper by Dr Heffernan, a naturalized German. This could well have been the result of a reference again. Possibly it led her to have hopes of snaring fatter game than Cotton. Heffernan lived at 7, Whitworth Terrace, a continuation of Spennymoor's main street. The two-storeyed house is still there, with a shopfront now.

Mary Ann made a good impression at first: the house was kept tidy, she seemed to be competent and the doctor was quite satisfied. Again she played the lady and got help with much of the cleaning. She is said to have paid for this in kind with provisions from the doctor's pantry. She mentioned to an acquaintance that she had not been used to hard work. She had access to the surgery so it was possible for her to steal arsenic. After her trial it was said that she had begun to poison Heffernan, who became suspicious and dismissed her. There is no evidence of this or that the police questioned Heffernan. She left the doctor and Spennymoor in June 1870. Shortly afterwards Heffernan found that a gold watch, guard and ring and some money were missing: suspicion, however, fell on his groom who was dismissed. There was comment that Mary Ann was immodest and immoral at Spennymoor and was fond of gaiety and dress to the extent of buying a silk dress to go to the races.

When she returned to North Walbottle in July, it appears Mary Ann presented herself first to Joseph and Frances Gallon – later witnesses to her marriage with Cotton. One can infer that there had been an emotional break with Cotton in the April and that she felt it was wise to have the help of the Gallons to renew the relationship. There could, of course, have been an understanding with Cotton that she would return to the hamlet after a decent interval. The day after her arrival she accompanied Joe Gallon and Fred Cotton into Newcastle and during the trip it was agreed that she should become Cotton's housekeeper.

Their bigamous marriage took place at the old church of St Andrew at the corner of Newgate Street and Gallowgate in Newcastle on 17th September, 1870. She was in about the same stage of pregnancy as when she married Robinson. Cotton gave his description as miner; his father was a labourer, but he had some schooling – he wrote his name well, clearly, carefully, with sloping letters. Mary Ann gave her 'condition' as widow, and it was entered that both lived in the parish.

So there was a new Mrs Cotton at High Pit. I have been told locally that she lived probably in Chapel Row or Coronation Row – stone-built back-to-back houses pulled down after the last war when the Coronation Pit was worked out, although their concrete floors remain. Apart from the pit-head Mary Ann would have wide country views all around. But Charles Cotton in his letter to Sergeant Hutchinson in 1872 mentioned a definite address. He said that Frederick Cotton and his first wife lived at 5, Devon Row, Walbottle Colliery.

A few weeks after the marriage Mary Ann filled in a proposal form to insure Cotton's two boys with the Prudential: the policy, however, was in Frederick Cotton's name.

It seems that she never settled at North Walbottle. The small community – the smallest in which she lived – would lack the variety of Spennymoor, never mind Sunderland. Her child, a boy, christened Robert Robson after her brother, was born in January, 1871, and this, so soon after the marriage, is said to have drained what patience the neighbours had for her. The tale that, after a row with a family, she poisoned their pigs probably originated here.

A resident of Walbottle told me that his grandmother ran to a farm for milk for Mary Ann, and that she remembered her as a pleasant, clean and generous woman who would give her an apple. But, as in other places, her name was used later to frighten children into obedience.

The Cottons left the area in the first half of 1871, probably in the spring. It is possible that they went to East Rainton before going on to West Auckland. The unfortunate Frederick Cotton seems to have made little impression on Mary Ann: she scarcely referred to him later.

She never wanted children for their own sake. Surely one can assume that. If she could have had her love-making without child-bearing, perhaps she would never have thought of poisoning.

CHAPTER FIVE

The Durham Spring Assizes:

March, 1873

Rumours were right. The Attorney-General for England, Sir John Duke Coleridge, appointed Charles Russell to lead for the prosecution. County Durham was a county palatine with its own Attorney-General, the Recorder of Liverpool, Mr Aspinall, Q.C., but he was by-passed.

Russell, an Irish Catholic and nationalist, forty years old, had taken silk the year previously – for a decade he made £10,000 or so a year. Authoritative, determined, often vehement, he came to be regarded as the greatest advocate of his time. He was twice Attorney-General under Gladstone, was raised to the peerage in his early sixties, and became Lord Chief Justice. Against Mary Ann he had the assistance of Mr Greenhow, Recorder for Berwick; Gainford Bruce; and H. J. Trotter.

On Monday morning, 3rd March, the Canadian-born judge, Sir Thomas Dickson Archibald, knighted a month earlier, said he intended to take the first case the next day. Russell asked if it might not be taken earlier than Thursday; also, he said, it was improbable that counsel would be instructed to defend the prisoner, and would his Lordship assign some counsel.

Mary Ann had asked that the letter from Charles Murray, handed to her in the Bishop Auckland court, should be passed to Lowrey, and he may have seen it, but it was in Smith's possession the same day. Murray's letter dated Monday, 24th February, 1873 was to George Hedley:

> If you will be good enough to place Mrs Cotton's friends in communication with me *at once*, (*say per return of post if possible*) I will take means to have this woman *well defended* by *able counsel* at the coming Durham Assizes.
>
> As the Durham Assizes are now near at hand no time must be lost. I must therefore hear from you or Mrs

Cotton's friends by Thursday morning the latest for it is requisite to have their sanction and assistance in getting up evidence on their behalf.

I am,
Yours truly,
Charles Murray.

Address for me
at *Box 54,*
Post Office,
Stockton-on-Tees.
Please place this note into the hands of Mrs Cotton's friends at once.

Smith replied immediately:

4, Gibbon Street,
Bishop Auckland.
25th Feby 1873.

Dear Sir

Regina v Cotton

Your letter of the 24th herein has been handed to me and I beg to inform you that I am defending Prisoner in the *first Case* viz for the murder of Charles Edward Cotton.

There are other Cases viz Natrass and the other children for which she is undefended.

She requests me to thank you for your offer and to say that she gladly accepts it.

Any assisstance or information I can give you will be at your service.

I might add that I have retained Mr Blackwell to defend in my Case.

yours truly
Geo. F. Smith.

Smith, as we know, never gave Blackwell instructions. One can surmise that his rejection of help in the vital first case also killed the efforts of the Bishop Auckland committee formed to help Mary Ann. The committee's solicitor, Thomas Labron, asked the Governor of Durham Gaol, Lieut.-Colonel Charles Armstrong, for permission to speak to Mary Ann. Armstrong provided him with a note:

27th Febr 73

Gatekeeper

Allow Mr Labron to see Mrs Cotton if she would like to see him.

C. Armstrong

Labron wrote on the note a message on his own to Mary Ann.

A Committee in Bp: Auckland are endeavouring to obtain funds for your defence at the ensuing Assizes and I am appointed as Solr. to such Committee and wish an interview should you have no objections.

So it was that on Monday, 3rd March, Mr Justice Archibald queried Russell:

'No one appears for the prisoner?'

'No, my lord,' replied Russell. 'The learned counsel who have been mentioned as likely to be instructed have received no communication.'

Russell's appointment over the head of Aspinall alarmed many, including members of the northern circuit. *The Times* said that considerable comment had been raised at the bar by the Government taking the case out of the hands of the prosecuting attorney and selecting four gentlemen, and that it had always been considered that without special patent the Attorney-General of England could not take precedence in the county over the Attorney-General for Durham: an indignity, wholly undeserved, had been cast upon Aspinall, whose experience in criminal matters was unsurpassed.

A special court of the northern circuit, held on Sunday, 2nd March, passed unanimously a resolution regretting that the Durham Attorney-General had not been given the case and trusted that, even now, her Majesty's Attorney General would meet their wishes.

In the House of Commons on the following Tuesday night a Mr Wheelhouse asked Mr Gladstone, the First Lord of the Treasury, whether steps would be at once taken to place the Attorney- and Solicitor-General of the County Palatine of Durham in the position to which they were rightfully entitled. Mr Gladstone said he had been endeavouring to ascertain what he could possibly have to do with the matter. This raised a laugh. He got another laugh when he said the matter belonged to those formidable mysteries of the legal profession into which he had never presumed to pry. The question, he said, ought to have been put to the Attorney-General.

The Attorney-General, however, replying to the northern circuit from Westminster Hall on Tuesday, 4th March, said that the matter of right had been decided by the Treasury. The excellent postal deliveries of the day are shown when he explains that he did not reply on the Monday because he wanted longer to consider a communication which he believed to be unprecedented. Mr Aspinall knew, he said, that it was through mere inadvertence that his services had not been called upon. The Treasury, however, did not admit that Mr Aspinall had the right to represent the Government in Durham; his office was intended as an honour only. He disclaimed any intentional offence, but did not feel he could withdraw the briefs. Sir John sent a copy of this letter to *The Times*.

There was no competition to be defence counsel. At lunchtime on Monday at the request of Mr Justice Archibald, Campbell Foster agreed to undertake the task – a Mr Part of the home circuit assisted him – and in the afternoon the judge announced that Regina v Cotton would begin on Wednesday morning. Russell and Campbell Foster decided that the first case – it was to be the only one – would be that of Charles Edward Cotton.

Thomas Campbell Foster, a Leeds man, was twenty years older than Russell. A legal writer and shorthand expert, he was an experienced member of the northern circuit. He was to take silk in 1875, and in 1879 was leading counsel for the crown at the trial of Charles Peace at Leeds.

It was the briefest of journeys this time for Mary Ann from the gaol to the adjacent Assize Crown court. The courtroom was crowded before ten o'clock; admission was for the most part by ticket, issued by direction of the Under Sheriff. Ladies of the county and city sat in the Grand Jury gallery, and very important ladies and gentlemen even sat on the Bench, the High Sheriff of the county, Colonel Surtees, being next to Mr Justice Archibald. Many lawyers were there for the opening. Hundreds of people were outside and many remained there for hours.

Mary Ann was brought in a few minutes before ten: two of her warders were women. She was placed in the front of the dock and there was gaped at. There was no baby with her this time. She looked care-worn, depressed, pale, and much older than when she first appeared in court at Bishop Auckland. The change is seen in photographs taken at the time. At Bishop

Auckland her hair had been brushed back from her forehead; now it was brought forward almost over her eyebrows. Her attendants had remonstrated with her about this, saying her hair did not look so nice. She said she was doing it because of 'that man Detchon from Newcastle'. (Detchon, however, was not called at the assizes). Mary Ann's black gown and black and white shawl were well-worn now and her small black bonnet looked a poor thing. She appeared to have the assistance of a crutch or stick and with it she gave a little quick hop to her front place.

After Campbell Foster had spoken to her she was given a seat. She rose from it to plead not guilty in a low, firm voice. During the day she scanned the face of each new witness, and kept her gaze away from the public.

Russell said the boy had been poisoned by his stepmother who had been formerly employed as a nurse at Sunderland infirmary. The household consisted of her husband, a collier; herself; Frederick Cotton junior and Charles Edward Cotton, sons of Cotton and stepsons of the prisoner; and Robert Robson Cotton, her son by Cotton. Afterwards there were lodgers, George and William Taylor, but they had left before the death of Charles Edward.

By July, 1872, she was in a state that was miserable enough. She was badly-off and had been left ill-provided for. Charles Edward was her only remaining child, but, having him to care and provide for, she was not able to earn her livelihood by nursing. She was a skilful nurse and, he believed, possessed considerable energy, cleverness and ability. She received poor law relief, but for some reason, which had not been clearly explained, she thought that this would be withdrawn. A child of the age of Charles Edward was not able to contribute to his own support, but was a tie and burden on the mother. She seemed to have done her best to keep the child decently clean, and if it had an insufficiency of food it was owing more to her misfortune than her fault. There was evidence that she cruelly and badly used the child, using great violence for its size and age and strength, and acted so harshly that they – the jury – would probably come to the conclusion that she had no love for it.

The child was insured by the Prudential Assurance office for some £8. About the 6th or 7th July he became ill: his step-mother gave him all he took. At her instance Dr Kilburn was called in. The child suffered from vomiting and purging, and the wretched life of the little creature ebbed away until it died on 12th July.

Russell then told of Kilburn's withholding of a death certificate; of his inconclusive post-mortem examination; and of the coroner's jury's return of death by natural causes because the doctor could not rule out such a possibility. He criticized the coroner and his jury for not suggesting skilled examination of the contents of the stomach. He told of Kilburn's later application of the Reinsch test; of the detection of arsenic; of the arrest; and of Scattergood's 'clear and undoubted' conclusions.

Could the child have been killed by poison taken or administered accidentally? At this point, he said, with the sanction of the judge, he should offer extensive evidence. He anticipated there might be an objection and would do no more now than indicate the evidence.

'I have told you', he said, 'that three children and the husband . . .'

Campbell Foster got to his feet. Mr Justice Archibald said to Russell, 'You have done enough: leave the details.'

This was the first indication of an issue which was to cause lingering dissatisfaction – the admissibility of evidence about other deaths in the household.

Russell said that the presence of poison in all the various organs showed that it could not have been given accidentally, but must have been administered over at least two or three days to work its deadly mischief. By whose mind and hand? The evidence on this point would be mainly circumstantial. This was a crime of a mind deliberately plotting, working out a plan secretly, in security, in darkness. Had the person charged the opportunity of getting poison? There was no arsenic in the prisoner's house when it was searched. But six weeks before the death of the child, Mrs Cotton sent the child itself, openly, to get two or three pennyworth of soft soap and arsenic. The West Auckland druggist refused to give it to the child and said that the prisoner should come for it herself. She then sent Mary Dodds, a neighbour and charwoman, for it. The mixture contained many grains of arsenic – he thought half an ounce; three grains would kill an adult. Half of the mixture was applied to some iron bedsteads which contained bugs. He was not saying that the remainder of the arsenic had been used to cause the death of the child; but the evidence showed the facility with which poison could be obtained. It was a simple thing to dissolve the mixture in water, when the arsenic would fall to the bottom.

Russell then came to motive. To a mind depraved, or morally weak, to one with a fancied sense of security, who could say what motive might not be adequate? There was some small pecuniary motive. There was the irksome tie of a child not of her flesh and blood. There was the feeling of poverty. The prisoner had some motive; had the opportunity – no one else had either.

The first witness, Isabella Smith, had been a nurse with Mary Ann at the old infirmary in Sunderland. Like other nurses, she said, prisoner had access to the surgery at any time. She had been at the infirmary on the day Mary Ann went to marry George Ward. Some three years later she had seen her again at the new infirmary when her name was Robinson, but Mary Ann had not been nursing then.

Questioned by Campbell Foster, Isabella Smith said that medicines were left made up in the surgery with the patient's name on them, and during the twenty-six years she had worked there she could go to the surgery when she liked. There was not always a surgeon there. No scientific training was given about poisons. It did not require much scientific knowledge to be a nurse, although they should know more than how to tuck people in bed or to give them broth.

Sarah Smith was questioned next. Answering Gainford Bruce, she told of the succession of deaths. Campbell Foster objected unsuccessfully, saying it was not proper to try the case by a sidewind. Later, in addressing the jury, he said both the Smiths were witnesses of prejudice. Sarah Smith said that the night before Charles Edward died he was very ill and seemed to be in a great deal of pain, and she said to Mrs Cotton that he was held very like his brother Freddy. Mrs Cotton had said: 'Yes, they are both alike. They are both one way.' To Campbell Foster she said people gossiped a good deal in West Auckland.

Mary Ann Dodds, who had lived next door to Mary Ann in Johnson Terrace, examined by Greenhow, said Mrs Cotton employed her to clean her house. Charles Edward had been a particularly fine little boy for going errands or anything of that kind: he was quite active and healthy. On Monday, 8th July, Mrs Cotton called the doctor herself, and Mr Chalmers arrived about midday. On the Friday morning, about twenty past six, a man came to her house and asked her to go to the prisoner's as the boy had died half an hour before. The child was on the sofa. Mrs Cotton said she thought it had died from gastric fever, and that it had started to take convulsion fits about midnight. She – Mrs Dodds washed and laid out the child. About a week before, prisoner said to her that she wasn't going to send the child to the workhouse, she would rather keep it, but they were going to take away the parish relief she got for it, and it would be hard for her to keep it for nothing. She had used nearly all the soft soap and arsenic mixture on the bedstead. The mixture had been sold in strong paper. What was left was put into a jug and left on a low sill in the lumber-room. (This jug or jar was never found).

In reply to Campbell Foster, Mrs Dodds said that as far as she could judge Mrs Cotton was kind to the boy. Russell got her to agree that it was a cruel and unfeeling act to remove the boy from the bed to the sofa the night before he died. Answering Campbell Foster, who later called her, 'a good old woman', Mrs Dodds said that the child was well-covered with bedclothes on the sofa. She had heard it said – it was 'a flying rumour' – that Mr Manning would marry Mrs Cotton but for the boy, but Mrs Cotton told her that this was untrue; Mr Manning did not object to the boy. She said Mrs Cotton's three rooms in Front Street, one above the other, were papered and carpeted, and that the room Mrs Cotton slept in with the child – the middle one – had green wallpaper: a green flower with a stone-coloured background. The green flowers were bright and fluffy. She had made about half-a-china-cupful of the soft soap and arsenic and had rubbed it into the joints of the bedstead and between the iron crossbelts under the bed.

The chemist and druggist, John Walton Townend, said the little boy – he didn't know his name at the time – asked for the soft soap and arsenic on 27th May. When he wouldn't serve him, Mrs Dodds came in five minutes or so later saying she had been sent by Mrs Cotton. The mixture he gave her would contain about half an ounce or an ounce of arsenic. The amount was entirely guesswork as he had been about to close his shop. He made a note of the sale in his pocket-book. Cross-examined by Campbell Foster, Townend admitted telling the magistrates that he mixed only from four to six grains. (Half an ounce is 240 grains. Russell had said three grains were sufficient to kill an adult). He said his was not the nearest chemist's to Mrs Cotton.

Thomas Riley, examined by Greenhow, gave his evidence of how Mary Ann had said she couldn't look after a smallpox case because of the boy; that the boy was also in the way of her marrying Quick-Manning; of how she had tried to get the boy into the workhouse; and of her observation that perhaps she wouldn't be troubled long as he would go like the rest of the Cottons.

To Campbell Foster he said there had been a great deal of gossip in the village about whether or not Quick-Manning would marry Mary Ann. He didn't remember anyone else wanting to send a child to the workhouse, but he had not known before of a boy left with a stepmother. He had informed the police not because of the gossip, but because of his suspicions about previous occurrences.

One of the relieving officers for Bishop Auckland, William Parr, said he had paid Mrs Cotton 1s. 6d. a week for the boy. At the last payment, on 6th July, Mrs Cotton had asked for the boy to be taken into the workhouse. He told her he could not do this. She said the boy was a great inconvenience to her; if it had not been for him she could earn ten or twelve shillings a week; he was not hers and she had no right to support him. Replying to Russell, Parr said the parish paid the boy's coffin money and to his Lordship he said he had not told Mrs Cotton that the 6th July payment would be her last: he had no instruction to say that.

The attitude of Mary Tate, Mary Ann's last cleaner woman, was even more hostile than it had been a week before. She said she was often in the prisoner's house washing and cleaning and that she had seen her ill-use the boy. She had told her to go canny, but Mrs Cotton had replied that the boy was hers. On Easter Sunday Mrs Smith had given a paste egg and an orange to the boy and he was crying for the orange which Mrs Cotton had put in her pocket. Mrs Cotton threw the orange into the fire. She said the egg and the orange would make him bad. The boy went on crying and Mrs Cotton then took a leather strap and thrashed him. When she started to do this, she, Mrs Tate, went upstairs to see Joseph Nattrass, the lodger, who was ill. (Mary Ann would be under some stress at the time. Her baby to Cotton was buried that day, and Nattrass was near to dying. The older boy had died three weeks previously).

Mrs Tate said she thought Charles Edward didn't get enough to eat. She had mentioned this once to Mrs Cotton who had told her that the Cottons were weak-stomached children and couldn't bear too much food. (Later that day Dr Kilburn said that the boy's body was wasted, with the belly distended). Some time before this, when Mrs Cotton got back from Newcastle where she had been to see her late husband's brother, she told the children that but for them she could get herself a comfortable home by marrying the brother. (Could there have been anything in this? Perhaps not, as the chance was there, surely, when only Charles Edward was left. But her feelings for Quick-Manning were dominant then – fatally for others – and also Cotton's brother could have moved to London: there was a brother Charles there at the time of the trial).

To Campbell Foster Mrs Tate explained that Mrs Cotton sometimes struck the boy over the ear and got hold of him by his hair. She could not say how often she had talked of this: the ill-treatment was a general topic. To Russell, she said, no, she had never whipped one of her children in a like manner, and the strap Mrs Cotton used was the kind pitmen wore round their waists.

A pitman, William Davison, said the boy was active but very white. He saw Mrs Cotton beating him on Saturday, 6th July, using a double belt of leather, 'for a canny bit', then stopping and starting again. The belt was called, 'a taws – a canny bit of strap used for the young uns. A good taws is a real useful thing,' he said. 'These Durham lads want it sometimes. A belt's a belt,' he added, 'and taws are taws.'

A pitman's wife, Mary Priestley, told of seeing Mary Ann striking and knocking the boy and of seeing her locking him both in, and out of, the house for long periods. She said she herself beat her five children in the right manner, with a single belt without a buckle: and she never took foot or knee to them.

Dr Kilburn said he was a member of the Royal College of Surgeons and he was called in by Mrs Cotton as he was passing the house about midday on the day before the boy died. He saw the boy again in the evening. The boy had been delicate-looking, but quite active. He had never had to attend him before, and he was startled to hear of his death. To Campbell Foster he said Chalmers had seen the boy previously. After making the post-mortem examination his own conclusion was that the boy had died from natural causes.

The doctor was then questioned by Campbell Foster about the poisons which had been prescribed: bismuth, hydrocyanic acid and morphia. Irritant poisons, he said, when taken in ordinary medical doses would not produce violent vomiting and purging. Their peculiar effects were shown chiefly on the coats of the stomach and intestines. Morphia sometimes brought on convulsive fits. There were four doses of the muriate of morphia in a white powder. Hydrocyanic acid was another name for prussic acid. It could be a formidable poison, but it was not an irritant. He used a preparation which contained four to five per cent of it. He put twelve doses into the bottle. Bismuth was an irritant poison: its effects were vomiting and purging if given in large doses, when it would act spasmodically. It caused inflammation of the gullet, stomach and intestinal canal. The three poisons prescribed were all strong and required great care in their administration.

Kilburn then agreed that Reinsch's process was sometimes objected to because of its uncertainty.

CAMPBELL FOSTER: You take a portion of the suspected substance with hydrochloric acid and boil it, and then place a piece of copperfoil in it. If the acid is not perfectly pure it may show traces of arsenic.

KILBURN: The acid I used was quite pure.

CAMPBELL FOSTER: You get the same appearance both from antimony and arsenic?

KILBURN: I did not try any other test.

MR JUSTICE ARCHIBALD: Do you mean it was a rough test as to whether it contained antimony or arsenic?

KILBURN: Yes.

To a further question from Campbell Foster he said, 'So far I was able to carry it, I left it uncertain whether it was arsenic or antimony.'

Kilburn said that arsenic was sometimes found in churchyards. He had sent some soil from the grave to Scattergood for examination. The viscera was buried on waste ground in his garden: he had not buried anything there before; the ground was not used as a rubbish place; it was a playground for his children.

Campbell Foster then turned to the green wallpaper. He asked Kilburn if he knew anything at all about these arsenical papers.

KILBURN: I have not seen any ill effects from them.

CAMPBELL FOSTER: You have seen them. They are bright green, are they not?

KILBURN: Some are.

CAMPBELL FOSTER: Fluffy and very handsome.

KILBURN: Yes.

The doctor agreed that arsenic threw off fumes with heat;

that a very hot fire in a small room could cause fumes to be thrown off. He amended this in his next answer which was to the judge, who asked what temperature would be necessary to throw off fumes.

KILBURN: I can't say exactly, but a very high temperature, not the temperature from a fireplace.

CAMPBELL FOSTER: Do not you know when the hydrogen test is being applied, if the person testing chances to breathe the fumes of the arsenic it is so deadly that death has arisen from it?

KILBURN: I do not know. I have not seen it all.

CAMPBELL FOSTER: Do you know that people have been attacked by chronic arsenical poisoning and some killed by living in rooms covered with paper in which arsenic has been employed?

KILBURN: I have heard so; but I should think it not very likely in these cases. It may cause suffusion of the eyes; irritation of the nostrils, and colic pain about the stomach, but I don't think it would produce death from a wallpaper.

CAMPBELL FOSTER: Do you know its effects in repeated instances have proved so injurious to health, and even fatal, that in Prussia it is prohibited?

KILBURN: I have heard of it.

JUDGE: (to Campbell Foster) Your question is very speculative, and can hardly be asked. Your cross-examination is of a very speculative character.

CAMPBELL FOSTER: (to Kilburn) Did you find the pulse of the child as high as 120?

KILBURN: Yes.

CAMPBELL FOSTER: That indicated heat – feverish heat?

KILBURN: Yes.

CAMPBELL FOSTER: Now, assuming the child was lying in that state of heat upon a mattress, which might have been turned after lying upon something like three quarters of an ounce of arsenic: the child might be impregnated with arsenic sleeping upon it. Would it be likely to imbibe anything that would be arsenically injurious?

KILBURN: I don't think so.

CAMPBELL FOSTER: Why not?

KILBURN: I don't think it would absorb sufficient.

CAMPBELL FOSTER: Do you know in regard to absorption, that there is an instance in the books where washing the hands with water impregnated with arsenic . . .

JUDGE: Put it whether from his general knowledge it would have such an effect.
CAMPBELL FOSTER: Do you know, from your general knowledge, that any person washing the hands in water impregnated with arsenic for curing some cutaneous disease, that that was sufficient to absorb arsenic enough to kill the person?
KILBURN: If the hands were chapped very much they might absorb sufficient.
JUDGE: If the skin was whole, how would it be then?
KILBURN: I don't think a person would absorb arsenic to do injury.

Kilburn agreed that the boy would be more susceptible to disease because he was delicate, and Campbell Foster concluded his cross-examination by obtaining assent that the doctor had found no marks or bruises: that there was no evidence on the body of the boy having been struck.

Russell re-examined on the wallpaper; the soil and the medicinal poisons. In reply Kilburn said he had not observed any arsenical green paper in Mary Ann's home. He believed such wallpaper was the most expensive because of the character of the colour. It took as much as 380 degrees of heat to give off fumes from arsenic, and the heat of the room would not exceed 60 or 80 degrees.

He said sometimes in cemeteries the clay had an arsenical taint, but the cases were rare.
RUSSELL: If a child was properly covered by linen and the ordinary grave clothes and enclosed in a coffin, would there be, in your opinion, any probability of any absorption?
KILBURN: I should think very little.
RUSSELL: Would there be, in your judgement, speaking as a scientific man, any chance whatever of absorption in the course of a few days?
KILBURN: No.

The doctor said the medicines he prescribed after his second visit were carefully compounded. These were the mixture of bismuth and hydrocyanic, to be taken every two hours, and the powders, each containing an eighth of a grain of morphia, to be taken night and morning, until the boy was relieved of vomiting.
RUSSELL: Would there be any possibility of injurious effects from the administration of such poisons in such doses?
KILBURN: None at all.
RUSSELL: Would doses of morphia in the quantity prescribed have any tendency to produce fits?

KILBURN: None.

Archibald Chalmers said he had been Kilburn's assistant for thirteen months. He buried the viscera in Kilburn's garden, on the east side, in some rather damp soil where there was no grass. On Monday, the 8th, on his first visit, the boy complained of pain over the stomach and bowels, sickness and some purging. He gave an effervescing mixture of bi-carbonate of soda and a few minims of prussic acid (two tablespoonfuls to be taken every two hours), and half a dozen powders of tartaric acid. There was no effect whatever. On the Wednesday the boy was worse and he gave him a mixture of bismuth, bi-carbonate of potass and prussic acid to be taken every four hours. It had not the slightest effect. Replying to the judge he said the mixture was quite safe to take; there were only a few minims of prussic acid.

CAMPBELL FOSTER: Were the poison bottles all on the same shelf in the surgery?

CHALMERS: They are kept separate on the second shelf from the top.

CAMPBELL FOSTER: How many will be there?

CHALMERS: Well, most of the strong poisons, such as arsenic in powder and solution – prussic acid, and the like.

CAMPBELL FOSTER: Now, you wanted bismuth. Was it on the same shelf?

CHALMERS: No, it was not. It was on the other side of the surgery.

CAMPBELL FOSTER: How far was the arsenic bottle from the prussic acid bottle?

CHALMERS: I can't say for certain, but it would be the fourth or fifth bottle on the shelf.

CAMPBELL FOSTER: Then which was the prussic acid bottle?

CHALMERS: Near the end of the shelf. There were eight or ten bottles on the shelf in all. It is a bottle containing fluid.

CAMPBELL FOSTER: Is there any solution of arsenic on the same shelf?

CHALMERS: No.

Chalmers had just said – although he could have been speaking generally – that arsenic in solution was kept on the shelf. One could infer, as Campbell Foster did, that arsenic in powder must certainly have been there. The evidence from Chalmers and Kilburn about the poison bottles was conflicting. Campbell Foster was to follow up the possibility that Chalmers had made a mistake in making-up a prescription: that he could have been distracted.

CAMPBELL FOSTER: Is Dr Kilburn what you call a parish doctor?

CHALMERS: I believe so.

CAMPBELL FOSTER: And a great many people would frequently call at the surgery for their medicine?

CHALMERS: Yes, there was always somebody waiting.

CAMPBELL FOSTER: Was there on the day you made the preparation for Cotton's child?

CHALMERS: Yes.

CAMPBELL FOSTER: And how long did they talk to you before they were supplied? Would it be an hour?

CHALMERS: Oh no, I would get what they wanted in ten minutes.

Chalmers said Mrs Cotton had seemed very anxious that he should see the boy, and that as far as he could judge showed all the kindness and attention which a mother ought to show. The boy never seemed to improve. He saw him three times: on the Monday, the Tuesday evening and the Wednesday.

Re-examined by Russell, Chalmers said he had been very much surprised at the boy's death. Before assisting Dr Kilburn he had served a five years' apprenticeship to a surgeon, followed by four years at Edinburgh University Medical School and he had considerable experience in compounding medicines: in fact, it was his business. All the poison bottles in the surgery were plainly and properly labelled and he was sure he had made up the prescriptions accurately. There had been nothing dangerous in the medicines he compounded, even for a child of tender years.

At half-past-five the court adjourned. Mary Ann had actually laughed, joining in the general merriment at some efforts of Mr Justice Archibald to understand the dialect. The jurors – all men were locked up at Mrs Carr's, the Half Moon Hotel, after being assured that the best attention would be paid to their comfort and convenience.

THE MIDDLE DAY: 6TH MARCH

On the Thursday morning the waiting jurymen put aside their morning papers as Mary Ann appeared, looking even paler and weaker than before.

Thomas Scattergood was the first new witness. He said that, after washing away black soil, he found the stomach red in patches and strongly inflamed by, in his judgement, an irritant poison. There was no food in the stomach, except small bits of onion skin. There was also 58/100ths of a grain of arsenic: this was from the fluid ounce which was all Kilburn sent on to him. There was more arsenic in the substance of the stomach, in the contents and substance of the bowels, in the liver, heart, lungs and kidneys. There was none in the spleen.

RUSSELL: Do the symptoms lead you to suppose that one or more doses were administered?

SCATTERGOOD: In my opinion, they point rather to repeated doses over several days. The presence of arsenic in the stomach implies recent administration. The quantity found is no indication of the quantity administered.

He said the moment arsenic was taken it began to be discharged: by vomiting; in urine; by laxity of the bowels; by absorption into the blood. All this indicated that a large quantity had been given. Two or three grains could kill a healthy adult; half of that would kill a healthy child of seven or eight. He found no morphia in the stomach, and a mere fraction of a grain of bismuth. The doctors' prescriptions would have no injurious effects.

Scattergood said arsenic and soft soap could be separated very easily by adding warm water, stirring, pouring off, and then repeating with cold water: pure white arsenic remained. He did this with a teaspoonful of the mixture in half a pint of water. Six grains of pure white arsenic remained and twelve grains were dissolved in the water. He said a teaspoonful or more of this water might be given to a child without the taste being noxious. There would be about 300 grains of arsenic in the mixture bought at the chemist's.

Answering Campbell Foster, he agreed that the green pigment in wallpaper contained a large amount of arsenic and that such papers were dangerous.

CAMPBELL FOSTER: Why, doctor?

SCATTERGOOD: Because a portion of this green substance wears off, or falls off, as the paper becomes dry, and it gets diffused with the air. Still more of it might be removed if the walls were swept or brushed in cleaning.

CAMPBELL FOSTER: That is exactly the answer I anticipated you would give. A sunbeam shining in through the window, doctor, would show the atoms or particles floating in the air.

SCATTERGOOD: Yes.
CAMPBELL FOSTER: Is that not the danger of these green papers that those in the room inhale these floating particles which may be the poison of arsenic?
SCATTERGOOD: It is said that persons have suffered in their health from that cause.
JUDGE: Have you ever known of death from that cause?
SCATTERGOOD: No, my lord, nor have I read of one.
He agreed that particles of dry arsenic could have fallen to the carpet from the bedstead, following getting in and out of bed, with the attrition of the crossbars over one another. If trodden on, it was possible that some might have risen in the air. The very gradual symptoms of poisoning then would be a cough; irritation of the air-tubes; thirst and inflammation of the eyes: but, he said, arsenic would not be found in the stomach. No, it might pass from the lungs into the blood and circulate through all the viscera and get into the substance of the stomach, but it would not get into the contents of the stomach that implied swallowing. 'A fatal case', he said, 'might occur from breathing in a room where there is a green paper, but I have never heard of one. I do not think that a sufficient quantity of arsenic could be floating about a room to cause death. Neither do I think that a sufficient quantity could drop from a mixture of soft soap and arsenic so that particles of it would float about to cause the death of a boy if he inhaled it.'
CAMPBELL FOSTER: When the boy was spinning his top, tossing his ball, playing at marbles, might he not have picked up two or three grains of arsenic?
SCATTERGOOD: No. Besides he could not very well spin his top in that room: there was a carpet on the floor. (Laughter).
CAMPBELL FOSTER: Now, you know that when a piece of bread falls to the floor, it always does so with the buttered side downwards? (More laughter).

Scattergood agreed with the possibility of some arsenic being picked up and swallowed in this way. He also said arsenic could be absorbed by broken skin. Questioned by Mr Justice Archibald he said he did not know of any fatal case following such absorption, and arsenic would not be found in the stomach. To Russell he said he did not attach any importance to the room having a green paper. The symptoms of the illness would have been quite different. There had been nothing said by Mr Campbell Foster to alter his judgement that the boy had died from arsenic which he had swallowed.

With Scattergood the issue of admissible evidence came to the fore and more or less remained there. Russell asked if he had had to make three chemical analyses in the other cases, and then said the prosecution would not press for such evidence if the judge had any serious doubts about it. 'Of course, if rejected, we would be relieved of any responsibility,' he said.

JUDGE: What you propose to tender is evidence in other depositions?

RUSSELL: Yes.

He said he proposed to tender it because Campbell Foster in his cross-examination had suggested accidental poisoning and also natural causes. Campbell Foster, objecting, said such evidence was not collateral; it would prejudice a fair trial, and would bring in issues which the prisoner would not be entitled to have explained by cross-examination. He also said that until the evidence was decided to be admissible the jury had nothing to do with it and should retire. Mr Justice Archibald said the evidence was the same as that given before the magistrates at Bishop Auckland: there was no authority or precedent for the jury to retire. He ruled that the discussion must be in open court.

His Lordship and Russell cited the Queen v. Geering and the Queen v. Garner as authorities. Campbell Foster referred to paragraphs in *Taylor on Evidence*, on the exclusion of collateral facts on the ground of irrelevance, and he cited Regina v. Holt in which, when evidence on a second count was inadmissible, conviction on the first count could not be sustained. He said that if the other cases were brought in they ought to be brought in fully, making this a trial of many issues.

The judge then retired to consult, 'his learned brother', Baron Pollock. Returning, he said he had looked into the cases of Geering and Garner, and he thought the evidence proposed to be tendered came entirely within the principles of those cases and that he ought to receive it.

RUSSELL: Your Lordship will reserve no question about it?

JUDGE: I reserve no question about it.

Campbell Foster asked if, as there were conflicting authorities, his Lordship would reserve a case for the Court of Criminal Appeal. Mr Justice Archibald said he must decline: his mind was made up in the matter.

Chief Baron Pollock knew of the prevalence of child murder. In the Friendly Societies Select Committee Report of 1854, he said, 'child murder for the sake of burial money prevailed to a fearful extent', and the number of instances where great suspicion existed was far greater than the number of cases coming before him. It was this report which suggested that no burial money should be paid unless a death certificate from a qualified practitioner was produced, or the body was viewed by a surgeon, and that there should be a limit on the total amount paid-out when a child was insured with a number of societies.

The Geering trial was at Lewes Summer Assizes of 1849, where Mary Ann Geering was on a charge of poisoning her husband with arsenic. For the purpose of proving that death was not accidental, evidence was admitted of arsenic being administered to her three sons a few months later: two of the sons died.

Following the ruling, Phoebe Robson gave her recollections of the illnesses and deaths of young Frederick, of the baby, and of Nattrass, including the horrific descriptions of the fits Nattrass suffered. She also mentioned that a Mrs McKieve had done Mary Ann's washing – taking it home – before Mary Tate.

William Taylor, a joiner living at Shildon, said he lodged at the prisoner's house from before Christmas of 1871. Shortly afterwards Nattrass came to lodge, and then his own brother, George. He hadn't noticed the symptoms of the two children who died. He used to go to work at five in the morning and got back at five in the evening. To Campbell Foster he said Mrs Cotton prepared his meals and he was never ill while he was there. He had coffee and bread for breakfast. They all had meals together when possible, eating from the same loaf and drinking out of the same pot. Nattrass was on the night-shift and they ate together at weekends. When Nattrass took ill he lay near a fireplace; previous to that they had shared a bed. He thought the prisoner had been very kind and attentive to Nattrass and he did not know of any quarrel between them. He had never heard of any bugs about the place, and knew nothing of her getting any stuff to rub on bedsteads.

To Greenhow, Taylor said he remained in the house about two months after Nattrass died. Mrs Cotton then got some woman in to fettle the beds and cook the food: at that time she was waiting on Mr Quick-Manning, the exciseman, and not so much at home.

William Taylor would have left about the time of the purchase of the arsenic and soft soap – just before or after. Perhaps at that time Mary Ann had determined to rid herself of the other two in the Front Street house – Taylor and the boy –

because of Quick-Manning, and then delayed the poisoning of the boy while she tried to accommodate him elsewhere, with a relative or in the workhouse.

George Taylor, a blacksmith of Shildon, said he had not taken any notice of the two children when they were ill. He had seen Nattrass stretching in a fit. To Campbell Foster, he said the prisoner had always been kind and attentive to the children and to Nattrass. She had seemed very fond of the baby and used to dangle and fondle it. He paid her 11s. a week, the same as his brother. She did their washing. He had not heard any complaints about bugs. (George Taylor left the house some three or four weeks before his brother, about the time of Mary Ann's move to the Front Street house and when she would know she was expecting Quick-Manning's child).

Evidence of the other cases continued with the calling of Dr Richardson, who said he had not expected for one moment that Nattrass would die. His pulse had improved greatly and Nattrass himself thought he was getting better. To Campbell Foster, Dr Richardson said Mrs Cotton had come to him urgently about Nattrass on 23rd March. She said the symptoms were the same as in a previous illness, so he prescribed medicines which had been effective then, including morphia. He visited Nattrass first on Tuesday, the 26th; saw him twice the next day and each day until he died – seven times in all. On the Wednesday morning he thought it was the boy, Charles Edward, who told him that Nattrass had had fits. Nattrass had told him that Mrs Cotton treated him very kindly: he had never heard him say a word against her. He had understood, from Mrs Cotton, that she and Nattrass were about to marry.

CAMPBELL FOSTER: Then she lost a husband as well as a lodger.

Richardson said he still retained the opinion that Nattrass had a disease of the kidneys – Bright's disease. But it was not likely to cause death in two or three days. The kidneys performed their office too well, fetching out that which should not be brought out, and he did not know of an instance of cure when it was running its course. He affirmed to Mr Justice Archibald that his impression was that Nattrass died of Bright's disease. He believed he put typhoid fever on the certificate, with disease of the kidneys.

Replying to Campbell Foster, Richardson said he would not be much afraid if he had to sleep in a sheet washed with soft soap and arsenic, but he should not like it.

Dr Kilburn was re-called. He said in the case of young Frederick Cotton he gave a certificate of death from enteric fever. The symptoms of the baby, Robert Robson Cotton, were different: there was no vomiting or pain in the bowels, but feverishness, resulting, he thought, from teething trouble. The child died about nine o'clock at night: in the morning he had been lively and well, dancing and prattling on his mother's knee. His certificate was that death was due to convulsions after teething. The prisoner seemed to be very fond of the baby: he thought she had been kind to the children. He had no suspicion of foul play. Kilburn said the four graves were near to each other and soil from each was sent to Scattergood. Seven medical gentlemen were present at the exhumation of the two children.

Details of the other cases continued: from Sergeant Hutchinson, about the bottles, plates and parcels; from Dr Chalmers and from Dr Scattergood, who said in all three cases it was his undoubted opinion that death was caused by swallowing arsenic. Kilburn, again recalled, said it was now his opinion too, that swallowing arsenic had brought about the deaths.

At that Russell closed the case for the prosecution, whereupon Mr Justice Archibald pointed out that he had not given any evidence about the prisoner being in possession of arsenic at the time of Charles Edward's death. What evidence was there, asked the judge? Russell said he did not think a stronger case of circumstantial evidence could be made out. He had described means of getting arsenic. There had been the actual possession of a considerable amount. But that, remarked the judge, was six weeks before the death of the boy. He repeated his question: had Russell any evidence of the possession of arsenic about the time of death? Russell then said he could bring forward evidence that Mary Ann was in possession of arsenic at the time of the other deaths.

CAMPBELL FOSTER: But my learned friend has closed his case, and he cannot open it again.

JUDGE: If Mr Russell has any evidence showing that the prisoner was in possession of poisons at the time of the deaths, I think he should be permitted to call it.

It would be a dangerous and alarming thing, Russell said, if a case of the strongest circumstantial nature was to be considered doubtful because there was no direct evidence of the possession of poison. The witness who could have spoken, Jane Hedley, had unfortunately been taken in labour that very afternoon in the city. Her deposition, he was bound to say, was taken in the case of Nattrass only, and not in the case now before them. Mr Justice Archibald remarked that that would hardly do. Russell said a further deposition could be taken the next day, but that would mean postponing the case, and it was not worth that. No evidence, he said, of the possession of poison at the time of the boy's death existed. It was all a matter for the jury. Even if there had been no evidence of Mrs Cotton's ever being in possession of poison he would still have put the case to the jury.

Campbell Foster then asked Mr Justice Archibald to strike out the whole of the evidence tendered in the other three cases, as possession of poison previous to the deaths had not been shown.

RUSSELL: The proof of the possession of poison has nothing to do with the admission of the evidence.

Mr Justice Archibald said, on the principle of the Geering case, the prosecution was entitled to show the history of others in the house when under the same circumstances they had died of poisoning. This was to meet the suggestion that the death of Charles Edward was accidental. Campbell Foster retorted that he did not see how the analyses of Scattergood came into this. The judge said that at one time there had been an indication that the defence was going for natural causes. That was the opinion of the doctors, said Campbell Foster. He reiterated that it had not been shown Mary Ann was in the possession of arsenic when the other three persons died; there were other people living in the house at the time: the evidence should not be accepted. He concluded: 'I may now state that I have no witnesses to call.'

The court then adjourned. The jurors were locked up again in the Half Moon Hotel.

END DAY

Before she was taken up to the court the next morning Mary Ann expressed her fears that, because she was not paying full fees to her counsel, there could be neglect. Those about her calmed her somewhat with assurances that this would not be so. Occasionally during the day she rose from her front seat to speak to Campbell Foster. During Russell's address her lips quivered and she kept glancing at judge and jury. She was depressed, too, with forebodings because it was a Friday. Charles Edward had died on a Friday; it had been a Friday in August when she had been committed for trial for causing his death, and on the Friday a fortnight before she had been committed for the murder of Nattrass. *The Times* said the gallery was completely filled with ladies, and that Mary Ann, 'a comely-looking, gentle-eyed woman', seemed very anxious.

Mr Justice Archibald opened the proceedings by referring to the exchanges the previous evening. He said that when he made his observation on the indirect evidence he had the impression that Mr Russell would have laid before them evidence as to the actual possession of poison. It had been a misapprehension on his part. He thought, however, that the indirect evidence given was within the limits.

Russell said that the prosecution had not thought it fair to go further than they did.

It was said that Russell in his opening and closing addresses spoke with a power and earnestness that affected all within reach of his voice, and that at times he showed emotion that was something more than a rhetorical trick. It was doubtful, wrote, 'One in Court', whether a more able piece of pleading had ever been heard in the northern circuit, and his addresses justified the extravagant expectations of his hearers.

Russell said this was a case of direct and deliberate administration of poison. The object of the admitted evidence of the other cases was not to try the prisoner on all four charges; not to enable the prosecution to show in one case that the prisoner had murdered somebody else – this would not be fair, and the law would not allow it. But the law said that where there were a number of very similar occurrences in which the conditions, circumstances, symptoms, were much the same, then such evidence was properly admissible in enquiring into the death of any one of those persons. When suggestions were made that death was by natural causes, or by poison accidentally taken, then the law permitted this evidence to be given to negative these suggestions. The prosecution were entitled to prove if they could, that more deaths occurred under similar circumstances.

He said he would not dwell upon the strange early history of the woman, although there was the significant fact of her being a nurse at Sunderland infirmary where she acquired considerable skill in the administration of medicine and drugs, and perhaps some knowledge of the character of drugs, the uses to which they might be applied, and the circumstances under which they might be given.

He told of the death of Frederick Cotton, then of the two children and Nattrass within the space of three weeks. On 6th July, 1872, the once numerous household had dwindled down to only the prisoner and her stepson, Charles Edward Cotton. The child of seven was face to face with a woman, not his mother, who showed no signs of a motherly tenderness towards him. To her he was a tie she would readily have got rid of. But the joyless character of the boy's life, never warmed by the sunshine of a mother's love, could not entirely stamp out that spontaneous joyfulness which nature implanted in him. So on 6th July he was seen well, as likely as any boy in his position to grow strong as he grew in years. On that very day, when the prisoner complained that the boy could not be taken into the workhouse, and that she was afraid that the poor law relief would be stopped, this healthy child took ill. Before seven days had passed – to the surprise of everybody – he was dead: his young life snapped as a blasted, withered blossom.

They had heard Dr Kilburn's evidence as to what he stated at the coroner's inquest, and the view which he doubtingly and with hesitation then took. They might think Dr Kilburn should have suggested an analytical examination to the jury. The doctor gave his evidence like a man painfully anxious to tell the truth, and when they considered his position in a village society, how fearful was the responsibility of suggesting that there had been foul play! They would not be surprised that it required a man of greater decision and resolution to give expression to the doubts. The inquest had scarcely been held when these doubts came back with greater force upon Dr Kilburn, and he tried a test and came to the conclusion that there had been foul play.

The symptoms in the other cases were precisely the same, except for those of the infant, where a still more fearful tale was to be told. Here they had seen the child entirely recovered in the morning, and that night violent convulsions had come on and the child had died.

Mr Scattergood had said in the case of Frederick Cotton, junior, he found one grain and seven hundredths of arsenic, one eightieth of a grain undissolved; in Robert Robson Cotton a small quantity of arsenic was found; in Nattrass as much as seventeen and three quarters grains; in the contents of the stomach alone of Charles Edward more than two grains were found, taking the proportion analysed in the nine drachms. One must conclude death was by poisoning, probably by doses repeated and extended over some time, by arsenic taken through the throat.

His learned friend had exhausted ingenuity in suggesting, without end almost, what he thought were consistent ways by which the arsenic might have got into the stomach. He would not treat any of these suggestions, however irrational, with anything like the slightest approach to levity. This was no case for levity.

Had the boy taken the arsenic accidentally? Could they give that serious consideration when, according to Mr Scattergood's evidence, repeated doses must have been taken over seven days? The suggestion that there might have been a mistake in making-up the prescription was a mere suggestion which in a desperate case was bound to be put, but which had no foundation in fact. As for washing the hands in arsenical water. Where was the arsenical water? It was an ingenious fiction. And arsenic absorbed through the skin would not find its way into the stomach. And arsenic particles floating about the room: Mr Scattergood said they would not cause death: they would not account for arsenic in the stomach. Fumes given off from the wallpaper: the lowest degree of necessary heat for this was 280, and there was opinion that it needed 380 degrees. Then the bread and butter theory. The boy got bread, but he thought it doubtful if he got much butter. If such bread had fallen on particles of arsenic which had dropped from the bedstead, Mr Scattergood had said that some slight particles might be taken up – that was just conceivable – but they would not do any mischief.

And then there were the three other cases. Did they believe they were accidental poisonings.

They were inquiring into the history of one of the most dangerous, one of the most appalling, one of the most atrocious crimes that ever disgraced this great county. They knew that in cases of this kind it was not possible to call upon an eye-witness who could say, 'I saw the deadly potion mixed, and I saw it administered.' No poisoning case he knew of had ever admitted of such a proof as that. It would be a sad thing for society, and an appalling statement, if it was suggested that crimes of this nature which made one's flesh creep and one's blood curdle were to go undetected because no one could be called to the witness box to say they had seen it done.

No one could have motive but the prisoner. This first took

the form of money: as far back as October, 1870, there was the proposal by the prisoner to insure the boy. Mr Justice Archibald intervened here, saying the proposer had been the husband. Russell explained that he was going to say the proposal was signed by the prisoner, but the child was not hers, and the policy was in the name of the father. He allowed that it might have been at Cotton's insistence that the policy was secured, but he was suggesting that it was in her mind in July, 1872, the benefit would come to her should the child die. The amount to be paid out increased as the child grew up; it was not limited to cover funeral expenses. Even if she had got the money, the parish would still have paid the burial expenses.

The child had been locked-out one day, locked-in another day; not systematically ill-treated, but often treated with considerable violence which had compelled observers to remonstrate. The prisoner had no love for the child, if she had no active hate. On the Saturday she was prophetic when she said to Riley, 'He will go like the rest: he will not get up.' The following Friday the boy was a corpse. There was no prophecy so sure of coming true as one in which the prophet has in her own hands the means of realizing it. The boy did not 'get up'.

During the illness, the prisoner seemed to act with concern and anxiety, and she had called the doctor. Let them give that its fair weight, and no more. Such conduct was what they would expect from an innocent person; equally it was what they would expect from a guilty one. How damning it would have been if she had not called in the doctor: and what a bungler she would have been if she had not shown anxiety! It was the conduct they would expect from a designing person.

She knew that medical men had failed to discover the true cause of death in the three other cases, and she knew that a doctor would hesitate long before voicing suspicion against his own patient. She might have had, he said, some fancied, or real, sense of security.

She had got the poison openly six weeks before the death of the child. She had the means, the motive and the opportunity of administering the poison – no one else had. Was this a case in which they could be led to any other conclusion than the guilt of the prisoner? If they had no real, serious, or substantial doubt, then the law did not allow them, justice did not allow them, no consideration of good sense allowed them, to raise for themselves unreal, shadowy, unsubstantial doubts. Human laws did not require, human nature and judgement were not capable of, absolute certitude in these matters. If they approached this case with firm, upright minds and saw but one conclusion, then they must, as honest men, fearless of the consequences, looking neither to the right nor to the left, say, if such be their opinion, that this woman was guilty.

This closing address, on paper, seems adequate – as it was. It is surely doubtful that it was the most able piece of pleading heard on the northern circuit. The crucial importance of Scattergood is evident, and probably it was shrewd to dismiss quickly, almost out of hand, points such as a prescription making-up error and the bread and butter theory.

Campbell Foster then addressed the jury. He said there was nothing which could show that the prisoner had administered poison. The case had been discussed in the newspapers, and, as if that was not enough, there had been admitted into it matters which had nothing to do with it. The responsibility for that was his Lordship's, and any one who knew what it was to do an act of grave responsibility, knew the careful thought and anxious consideration with which the step had been taken. From the very first, before it was known that it could be admitted, evidence was given about the prisoner's past. He objected to it then, when Sarah Smith and Mrs Dodds gave evidence which had nothing to do with the case. What was it to them that she was once called Mowbray, once called Ward, if it was not to insinuate that Mowbray and Ward had died, poisoned by unfair means, and probably Cotton also? Mr Justice Archibald observed there had been no insinuation about Mowbray: insinuation had not been the object at all.

Campbell Foster said that the evidence of the other cases was to attempt to show that it was unlikely that arsenic had been given accidentally. If the prisoner had been tried and found guilty of the three murders, the law would not have allowed evidence of them to be put before a jury. She had not been tried, and yet it had been put before them. This was to prejudice them, to bias them, so that if they had doubt it would weigh against her. His learned friend could not walk alone; he wanted a crutch to help him. Would the Taylors, living in the house at the time, have lived there a day longer if they had suspected anything?

The prosecution had said that it was possible that the prisoner had got poison for the other cases in West Auckland, or elsewhere. Where was the chemist to prove it? Did they believe, with newspapers circulating up and down, that if poison had been sold a chemist would not have given information to the police by now? No chemist had come forward. The prosecution said she was guilty of those three deaths because she had poison brought into the house at a later date. And what about motives for the other deaths?

RUSSELL: I could not have done that.

JUDGE: It would not have been admissible.

There was no motive, Campbell Foster said. She had a direct interest the other way. She lived by lodgers. Nattrass was her lodger. And more . . . they were engaged to marry. (Mary Ann was said to have smiled here a little). Nattrass, said Campbell Foster, was earning good wages, able to keep her. Could a woman have a stronger motive to preserve his life?

His learned friend had insinuated that she poisoned her own infant, fourteen-month-old Robert Robson Cotton. One almost revolted at such a picture. A mother poisoning her own child! A mother nursing it, calling in the doctor, dancing it upon her knee, looking fondly at it, listening to its prattle, seeing its pretty smiles, while she knew she had given it arsenic, making its limbs writhe as it looked into her face wanting support and protection! (Mary Ann, understandably, began to cry). Depend upon it, said Campbell Foster, a mother could do nothing of that kind. A mother do that? They knew a mother's instincts. But his learned friend said she had poisoned this child. What motive? What had she to gain by its death? Was the infant in her way?

His friend said sending for the doctor was consistent with innocence. So it was. This woman knew that poison could be detected; and yet she had sent for the doctors. She had called in the doctors in all three cases. She was kind to the sick, she nursed them. How much of all this supposition rested upon the gossip of the old women who were called one after another and who tried to make three black crows out of one? The charges of cruelty had completely broken down. It had been no more than chastisement, and everyone of the three or four gossiping women had a belt, a whip, or a taws for her own children. it might be that there were curious and suspicious circumstances and some matters unexplained, but why put in these cases except to warp their minds? If his learned friend was justified in bringing forward the cases, it was a scandal to the law. Would they consider the case itself, irrespective of this lumber it had been made to carry?

It was a fact that papers printed with what was called

arsenical green, produced ill-health. It was certain that the fluff – the raised portion – got rubbed off, fell upon the ground, floated in the air. It could not be seen unless there was sunlight in the room, and then you saw myriads. It was these things, getting into the nostrils, down the throat and into the lungs, which produced illness – arsenical poisoning had been caused by such.

Then Mr Townend, the chemist, said there might have been 300 grains of arsenic among the soap. Where did all that go? It was in the room, spread upon the bed – 300 grains. It fell as it dried and was stirred every time anyone went into the room. When the boy played, a cloud of these poisonous atoms must have arisen and been inhaled: much would adhere to the tongue and nose and throat and be swallowed. It was no invention about the bugs – they were there. After the treatment of the bedstead what was left of the mixture was put in a jug. Assume that the jug was washed out imperfectly and then that the boy had a drink of water or milk out of it. Dr Scattergood had said it needed four or five rinsings. That would account for the grains in his stomach.

He did not say the boy died because the bedclothes were washed in arsenic and water, or because he might have washed his hands in arsenic and water, or that he inhaled arsenic, or drank it out of a jug, or because his bread and butter fell upon the floor: but he put these suggestions before them as suppositions by which the injury could have been done. Bismuth, prussic acid and morphia had been given: these might have produced the appearance of the stomach. It was possible that Dr Chalmers might have put in arsenic instead of bismuth – the grains were both white: the most careful chemists made mistakes. All these suggestions were fair and reasonable.

They should come to the conclusion that the prisoner was not the cold-blooded fiend who would administer poison to her child, watch the effect upon it while she pretended to nurse it. He did not understand such a thing. He could not believe it. They should try her as they would others. They should try her without these suspicions. They should not balance the evidence by taking prejudice into consideration and say the woman was guilty.

Campbell Foster's address lasted nearly two hours and at the end of it a Dr Hardy of Byers Green, standing in the reporters' box, applauded. Mr Justice Archibald rebuked him for this 'indecent manifestation,' and said he had a good mind

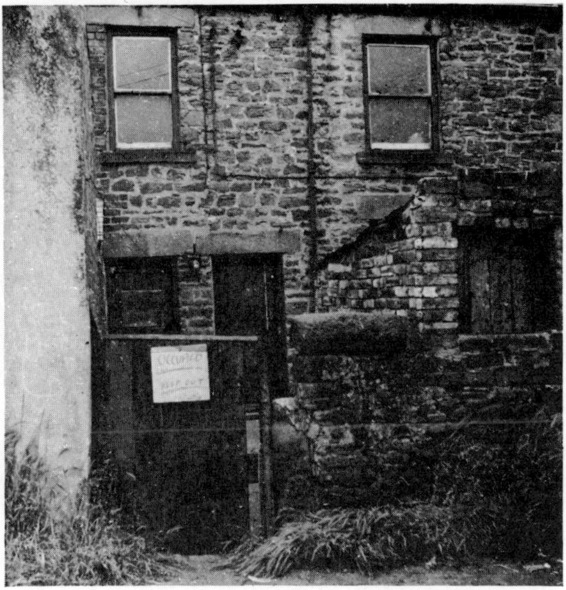

The back of Johnson Terrace. A passageway from the door on the left, No. 20, led to the front half of the back-to-back dwelling.

Frontage of Durham gaol and assize courts.

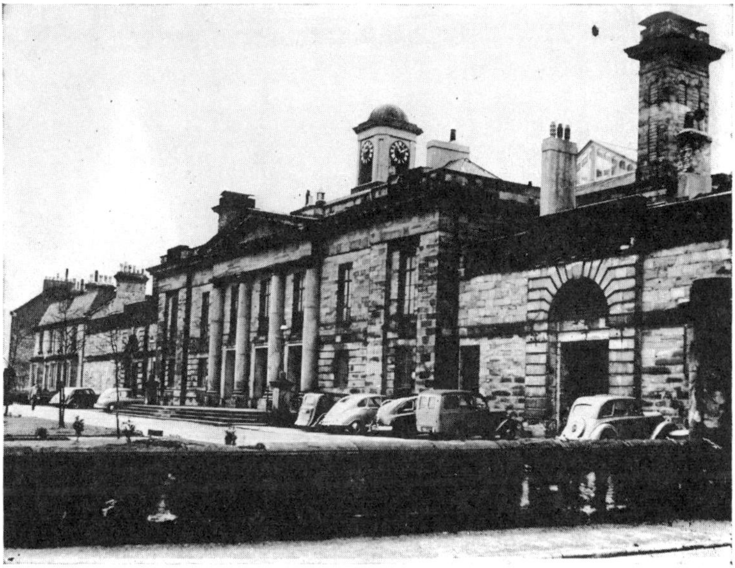

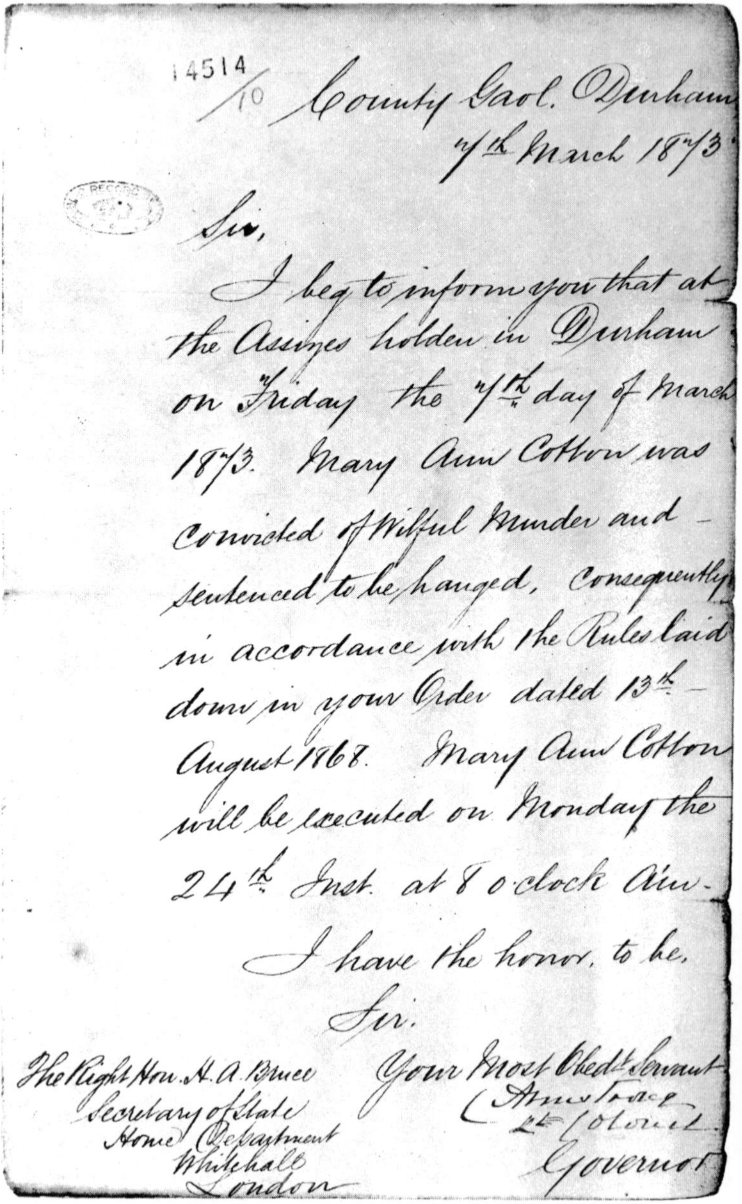

14514

10

County Gaol. Durham
7th March 1873.

Sir,

I beg to inform you that at the Assizes holden in Durham on Friday the 7th day of March 1873. Mary Ann Cotton was convicted of Wilful Murder and sentenced to be hanged, consequently in accordance with the Rules laid down in your Order dated 13th August 1868. Mary Ann Cotton will be executed on Monday the 24th Inst. at 8 o clock Am.

I have the honor, to be,
Sir,
Your Most Obedt Servant
C Armstrong
Lt Colonel
Governor

The Right Hon. H. A. Bruce
Secretary of State
Home Department
Whitehall
London

The Governor of Durham gaol to the Home Secretary.

to commit him to prison, as the offence was aggravated by being committed almost on the very Bench itself. Dr Hardy winced and apologized, and the court adjourned for twenty minutes for refreshment.

In his charge which began at seven minutes to two, Mr Justice Archibald said the case had been laid before the jury most fairly by counsel for the prosecution. The crime of murder consisted in killing with malice aforethought. The law implied malice in a person so charged, and it was for that person to give such evidence or explanation as might tend to do away with that implication. If they found that the act of killing came home to the prisoner, the law would imply wilful malice: it would not be necessary for the prosecution to show it.

Although evidence was given every day for what was called, 'motive', the law did not take notice of motive. What the law regarded was intention. In many cases it was almost hopeless to arrive at the hidden motives of action. The law put no such burden on those who prosecuted in cases of crime. The existence of motive might be extremely material where there remained a doubt as to whether the act had been done or not, but it was not essential that evidence of motive should be given. If they were satisfied that there was deliberate intention to commit the act it was needless to inquire into the motive.

Over and over again it was impossible to furnish direct evidence of the commission of crime. There were many crimes, particularly the one charged against the prisoner, which were plotted and carried out in secrecy, and if the law were to require that there must be eye-witnesses, that you were to have direct ocular testimony, many persons guilty of such crimes would go unpunished. Nothing so unreasonable was required by law. What was required was evidence to produce a moral certainty such as could be acted upon by any reasonable man. If evidence amounted to that, juries were bound to act upon it. The evidence in this case – a great deal of it, the most important portion of it – was circumstantial or indirect. Circumstantial evidence was the result of the proof beyond dispute by direct evidence of certain facts, and the inferences that were fairly deducible from these facts. All they could do was to arrive at a certainty which excluded all reasonable doubt.

The doubt to which they were bound, by the mercy of the law, was not one founded upon whim, caprice or speculative theories, but one they could reasonably justify to themselves. It must be a doubt which they would give effect to in any other transaction in life. It must not be irrational, not an impulse. It must be their deliberate conviction. If there was such a doubt they should give the benefit of it to the prisoner.

They were to decide the case on the evidence, not on the suggestions of counsel. The collateral evidence had been admitted solely upon the point of whether the death was accidental or not. It had been admitted because counsel for the prisoner had set up the theory that the poison had been administered accidentally. If there had been only the single case they might have a doubt whether the poisoning was accidental or not, but the prosecution were entitled, when deaths occurred under similar circumstances, to refer to them. He took the entire grave responsibility of allowing the evidence to be given. Many eminent judges had allowed evidence of a similar kind in similar cases.

Mr Justice Archibald then reviewed the evidence and the points put forward by Campbell Foster. He referred often to Dr Scattergood, pointing out where his evidence had been against defence counsel's suggestions. Mr Scattergood had said that, if the arsenic had been inhaled or absorbed, the symptoms would have been quite different. He had implied that there had been repeated administrations of arsenic, with some administered shortly before death. If the poison had been taken unwittingly from the jug, nothing was more natural than that the jug should have been produced. It had not been produced.

The question was whether the poison had been taken accidentally or voluntarily, or had been administered wilfully. Could they consider that the other three deaths were accidental? The probabilities pointed very strongly the other way. That no fewer than four persons should die in succession in some accidental manner was a series of accidents going beyond the bounds of probability.

If they thought the arsenic was administered wilfully, who administered it? Only the prisoner could have administered the arsenic in the shape it had been given. No one else had access to the child. The prisoner had both the means and opportunity of administering the poison. Did she avail herself of these means and of the opportunity? No one saw her. If she gave the poison it must have been unknown to the patient, a secret process.

The conduct of the prisoner in one view was perfectly consistent with innocence, and upon another with hypocritical and deceitful conduct. If there was a reasonable doubt whether the prisoner administered the poison, they ought to give her the benefit of that conclusion and doubt. If they were impelled irresistibly by the evidence that it was the prisoner who administered the poison then they were bound to find her guilty.

When Mr Justice Archibald had ended his summing-up at twenty minutes to four a juryman indicated he would like to ask a question. 'It is a pity it was not asked before', observed the judge. The juryman, saying it had just occurred to him, asked if the same quantity of arsenic instead of bismuth had been used by mistake in the prescription, would the same amount of arsenic have been found in the body as was found?

Dr Kilburn, asked to answer this, said three drachms of bismuth were put in the prescription. There had been no white arsenic in powder in his surgery at the time: all the arsenic they had was in a fluid state.

This reply caused Campbell Foster to write to the *Newcastle Daily Chronicle* the next day. He said previous evidence, from Chalmers, had been that there was arsenic in powder on the main poison shelf, and that Kilburn had said that bismuth in the form of a sub-carbonate, also a white powder, was in a bottle on the same shelf. Chalmers, he said, had admitted that he was chatting to pauper patients as he made up the prescription.

There is no doubt at all that there was disagreement and conflicting evidence from Kilburn and Chalmers about what poisons they had and the disposition of the bottles.

The jury retired at ten minutes to four, and a bigamy case was started in the court. After nearly an hour there were loud whispers of, 'The jury.' The bigamy case was stopped and at sixteen minutes to five the jurymen were back in their places. Mary Ann re-appeared and clutched the dock-rail. Answering the Clerk of Arraigns the foreman of the jury, a Mr T. Greener of Darlington, said a verdict had been agreed upon.

'Do you find the prisoner, Mary Ann Cotton, guilty or not guilty?'

'Guilty.'

'As so you all say?'

'Yes.'

Mr Justice Archibald put on the black cap. The Clerk asked Mary Ann if she had anything to say why the sentence of death should not be passed upon her. She muttered a reply, and the judge asked what she had said. He was told she said she was not guilty.

The judge said:

'Mary Ann Cotton, you have been convicted, after a patient and careful trial, of the awful crime of murder. You have had the benefit of the assistance of counsel for your defence, and everything that could possibly be urged on your behalf has been said, but the jury have been led to the only conclusion to which they could have come – that you are guilty. You have been found guilty of the murder, by means of poisoning, of your stepson, whom it was your duty to cherish and take care of.

'You seem to have given way to that most awful of all delusions, which sometimes takes possession of persons wanting in proper moral and religious sense, that you could carry out your wicked designs without detection. But, whilst murder by poison is the most detestable of all crimes, and one at which human nature shudders, it is one the nature of which, in the order of God's providence, always leaves behind it complete and incontestable traces of guilt. Poisoning, as it were, in the very act of crime, writes an indelible record of guilt.

'In these last words I shall address to you, I would earnestly urge you to seek for your soul that only refuge which is left for you, in the mercy of God through the atonement of our Lord, Jesus Christ.

'It only remains for me to pass upon you the sentence of the law, which is that you will be taken from hence to the place from whence you came, and from thence to a place of execution, and there to be hanged by the neck until you are dead, and your body to be afterwards buried within the precincts of the gaol. And may the Lord have mercy upon your soul.'

Mary Ann sat down, a pallor gripping her face. The warders fussed about her as she seemed to be slipping into unconsciousness. They carried her down, insensible, or nearly so, to the waiting-room, where they brought her round.

Charles Russell spoke to the judge, proposing that the other indictments should be left upon the file: Mr Justice Archibald agreed. People, excited, left the court slowly. The bigamy case, resumed immediately, seemed to be held in a deserted room.

The governor of the gaol wrote to the Home Secretary,

County Gaol, Durham.
7th March 1873.

Sir,

I beg to inform you that at the Assizes holden in Durham on Friday the 7th day of March 1873 Mary Ann Cotton was convicted of wilful murder and sentenced to be hanged. Consequently in accordance with the Rules laid down in your Order dated 13th August 1868, Mary Ann Cotton will be executed on Monday the 24th inst. at 8 o'clock a.m.

I have the honor to be,
Sir,
Your Most Obedt Servant
C. Armstrong
Lt Colonel
Governor.

The Right Hon. H. A. Bruce,
Secretary of State
Home Department
Whitehall
London.

A similar letter, but not so coldly formal, was sent to the Home Secretary the next day by Richard Bowser, Under Sheriff for the county. He said it was, 'proposed to appoint Monday, the 24th inst. at 8 o'clock in the forenoon for her execution'.

CHAPTER SIX

The numbered days

Ther Will not be enny Mor Sunday schoule teaching for me now

With the custom of three Sundays intervening between sentence and death, to be sentenced late in the week meant that Mary Ann had less time to live than she might have had: fewer than seventeen days.

The women warders' retiring room had been turned over to her and her baby. Well-lit and with a good fire, it had in it the cradle, an iron bedstead, a table, two chairs and a stool. Usually two women prison officers were with her day and night.

She was said to be cold and reserved. She gave no indication at all that she was likely to confess. After the shock of the sentence she slept for a long time on the Friday night, and her appetite at first was good. She was respectful to the people about her, and in the main they considered her cunning as well as intelligent. In the long periods when she was withdrawn and looked calm she did not want to catch anyone's eye. But there were times when she did talk. She was most concerned to promote petitions for a reprieve.

Far away a file on her was nearing closure. The Treasury Solicitor wrote to the Hon. A. F. O. Liddell at the Home Office. 'I beg to inform you that the prisoner was convicted of wilful murder and was therefore ordered by Mr Justice Archibald to be hanged. I return the papers.'

On Monday Mary Ann wrote to George Moore, a Bishop Auckland wine and spirit merchant.

Durham County Gaol,
10th of March, 1873.

Sir,

I will take it as a great favour if you will call and see me at your earliest convenience. Will you please to ask Mr Labron to come with you. I wish to consult with you about

> getting me a petition for my life to be spared. You must get a Visiting Justice's order to come in, and you must tell him what your business is with me. Mr Fawcett, South Bailey, Durham, is one, and Mr J. F. Elliot, Elvet Hill, Durham, is another. Either of them will give you an order for me.
>
> Yours respectfully,
> M. A. Cotton.

The local newspapers said the handwriting was bold and good and showed that the prisoner had had a better education than was supposed. It is certain, however, that someone in the gaol wrote or drafted the letter for her. Moore, evidently at the head of the so-recently sympathetic businessmen in Bishop Auckland, had experienced a change of outlook, for he replied that he could not hold out any hope of a petition succeeding and trusted that she would avail herself of the short time she had to live by preparing to meet her Maker.

The morning after the verdict the *Newcastle Journal* spoke of a 'monster in human shape,' and of a 'series of crimes so inhuman with scarcely the motive or the temptation of the common thief'. Saying that there were twenty-two deaths mentioned in the police report, the paper continued,

> Murder grew with her. Perhaps the most astounding thought of all is that a woman could act thus without becoming horrible and repulsive. Mary Ann Cotton, on the contrary, seems to have possessed the faculty of getting a new husband whenever she wanted one. To her other children and her lodger, even when she was deliberately poisoning them, she is said to have maintained a rather kindly manner. We feel instinctively that the earth ought to be rid of her. Pity cannot be withheld, but it must be mingled with horror. The spectacle of a human being without natural affection is fearful. She has been a murderess out of heartlessness. She has killed off all that came in her way with much the same indifference. That she should give some signs of human kinship by experiencing the pangs of remorse are the best and kindest wishes that can be felt.

The *Durham County Advertiser* said,

> Such crimes are far more hideous than murders committed in the heat of passion; and it is strange and terrible that

> persons capable of committing them can maintain the quiet decencies of ordinary life. There was no hatred or passion, but a sort of diabolical inhumanity which made the woman absolutely indifferent to everything except the attainment of her own paltry ends. Perhaps the greatest wonder is that a woman could successfully practise for so many years a system of poisoning without betraying her dreadful secret. She had no difficulty in getting four men to marry her, and it is said to have been one of the reasons for wishing to get rid of her stepson that the child was an obstacle to her marriage with a fifth.

The *Northern Echo* said her successes made previous cases of poisoning seem insignificant, and that it was said that after one or two successes in administering poison a sort of fascination or mania took hold of the experimenter, and victims were struck down for hardly any motive beyond that of gratifying a morbid feeling.

The *Daily News* said that the full sickening narrative had been only partially heard. Other women had poisoned people they considered in their way, in the main, without obvious animosity. Mary Ann was another illustration of the remark, often made, that women had a natural turn for poisoning. There was no doubt that poisoning, usually by arsenic, was the most common of the serious crimes of which women were convicted. Women had been the most successful poisoners, detected only because their success had made them reckless. Perhaps the peace and quietness with which poisoning could be done gave the crime a charm in the eyes of women over other forms of murder.

The paper then said that the payment of even a small sum for every child that died was often a premium on neglect, and that they could wish that life insurance among the very poor might assume some form which had less the appearance of offering inducements, if not to murder, at least to neglect.

Thomas Riley was singled out as the person responsible for bringing Mary Ann to justice by his unwavering pressing for investigation.

On the Tuesday Colonel Armstrong came to Mary Ann's room and told her he had received confirmation of the execution day: her first intimation of the day. She said, 'Thank you, sir,' and she did not discuss the knowledge at first with her attendants.

She answered two letters that day. The *Newcastle Journal*

later gave them, 'verbatim et literatim', they said. The first was to an old neighbour.

March the 11

My der frend
I have just reseaved your letter which it will be to know youse to tell you the state of mind but ie must say As ie saide before i Am not guilty you know What i toald you Before When i Was At Auckland regarding the bodley child. But Smith has Lead me rong if he told me not to speake A single Worde if i Was Asked Ever so hard or Ever so mutch i Was not to say it was Wrong that Would be All don in durham, he has never Brote forth Won Witness fore me, he new What they Ware Wanted fore not only the childe but for my sealfe i do no Want nothing but the trouth of Every Won then ie Would have A Chance fore my Life. As fore Riley god Will juge him, not A orthely Juge. if it had not been for smith i should make 5 or 6 of them stand With thar toungs tyde And Would yet if ie could get repeaved to stand my other Tryeles. ie have wrote to Mister Labron the soliseter And to Mr. Mower spiret mearchent B A to see if they can get Me A portion up so i hope you Will do All you Can fore me. you can see them Enny time so fare Well, if We do not meeat on Earth I hope to meeat in heaven.
So far Well Write as soune As you Can
M A Cotton

No explanations, no rationalisation, no recital of detail of what might have been done in her defence, but an understandable feeling of bitterness against Smith, against neighbours who spoke against her, against the absence of others who might have spoken for her. One can be moved towards her; to wondering if it were possible for her to be unknowing: 'i do not Want nothing but the trouth of Every Won . . .' Or had she a feeling that whatever she had done was in accord with herself, was as it should be, justified, impossible to think about as being wrong? But there was not a word of sympathy for the dead.

The other letter, an impressive, flowing one, was to Henry Holdforth of Andrew Street, West Hartlepool, an old friend of the Robson family, who had been a fellow coal-miner and worshipper in Murton. He was eleven years older than Mary Ann.

March the 11

My der frend

i reseved your most kind And Welcome Letter this morning Whitch it hurt my feelings veery mutch you say you have read my case in the papers Well my der frend I hope you Will not Juge me rong As i have been on the Awfill crime of murder of Charles Edward Cotton Whitch i Am not guilty of it thoe to reade the evidence that comes in against me you may think i am but if ie must Tell you I am not guilty I have been miss Lead With a man thea call smith he took upon him to Looke after my case He told me not to speake a worde Let the witnesses say what thaye would I had not to speake it woulde be all don at durham and my evedens was niver given propley into the Counsler or I should not come to what i have for i had a first class Counsler to defend me but i should like if i could get a portison up to spare my Life you speake of mother, had i my mother i should not been hear, fore my father i have not seen him since mother death, that is 6 years 15th of this month, so he has no mor fealing now then he had when we had mother but thanke god she is i hope in heaven, she Left evry resons to beleaiv she Was happy my Dearly bloved Brother, father Robson, and my husbent W. Mowbray and if my Dear Child is there so i shall hope to meet them on the other side of Jordon the time you speak of my dark eyes i wos happy then, and them Wos days of joy to all of our soles but this Last 6 years my Life has been misreable for i married A Man they call James Robinson he had 3 sisters i never Wos Looked on as i should be With non of them he and i not Ergree We had sum Words Aboute sum money and i Left the house fore a few days I did not wish to part from him As i had no home i Went to south hetton stayed ther When i returned ther wos no home for me he had sold What he did not Want And tooke the othe things and Went to Live With his sister so i might go where i Liked so i got married to this Man Cotton he dide the Month After We come to Aucland to tell you All the past i can not As it is to hartrenden to think on i should Like if you could Write to gorge hall and do What you can fore me to be spared With my Life i have that faith to belieave if the trouth Wos told i should be sparde so i hope you Will do What you can for me As i have no frends to Looke After me nothing

But strangers What has only knone me A few month so i hope And trust in god you Will do All you Can And get gorge hall to do the same I do knot knone Whar to write to him so i must Come to A Close give my kind love to All that know me hoping they Will do the same so far Well i must say ther Will not be enny Mor Sunday schoule teaching for me now but i shall try to put my trust in god As you knone i Wons did And ther was non on Earth happyer then i wos then but He says he Will not Leave us in trouble he says if We Aske in faithe it shall be given in troubles i Will not leave th All Mine enemys Whispers together against me even against me do they imagine this evil So no mor from A frendless Woman no i may say is forsaken By the World, but I hope not by god.

M A Cotton

Let my fate be known to All that know me i hope meat All my frends in heavn.

Is she conditioned to act to the end? Her reference to her mother is in a manner which makes one doubt that she poisoned her. There is nostalgia for the so-lost innocent days of youth, flowing into free verse:

the time you speak of my dark eyes
i wos happy then
and them Wos days of joy
to all of our soles

and, 'ther was non on Earth happyer then i wos then.' There's the affectionate reference to the first of her husbands, although, even allowing for the custom of the time, the christian name initial points to an insulation, a separateness, perhaps an absence of real sentiment. And which child is the 'Dear Child'? Isabella Mowbray, who lived longest, until she was nine? Against this is the police asterisk alongside her name, although the police could have been much influenced by Mary Ann's first enemies – Robinson's sisters. There's the heart blow of not being able to resume life with Robinson: the feeling against him and what that exclusion led to; the dismissive reference to Cotton; the import of the line, 'to tell you All the past i can not As it is to hartrenden to think on.' There's the dissatisfaction with her stepfather, George Stott. And there's a fervent return to the religion of her youth, the increasing, desperate realization that what solace and support she can have is only there. The George Hall she mentions is thought to have been her sweetheart in Murton or South Hetton before she met Mowbray.

The first appeals for mercy came from London. On 8th March a Mr T. C. Huddleston of Kentish Town wrote to the Home Secretary hoping that Mary Ann would be examined to see if she was insane, and an H. Hale of Old Kent Road entreated that she should have the benefit of any extenuating circumstances.

On Wednesday, 12th March, she received her first visitor, Mrs Margaret Stott, who with her husband, John, brother of Mary Ann's stepfather, ran the Bridge public-house in South Hetton. Mrs Stott had a companion with her for her own support, Jane Stubbs. Mary Ann burst into tears when Colonel Armstrong brought the two women into the room. She said to Mrs Stott she wished her stepfather would come to see her, and she didn't understand why he hadn't done something for her as he had known her from childhood.

Mrs Stott asked her: 'Why did you do it?'

Mary Ann pointed to the cradle, 'I am as innocent of the crime as that baby. The only crime I'm guilty of is bigamy, but what was I to do when that man Robinson drove me to the door?'

She said she felt certain that Mr Bethune, minister of the old parish church at Seaham, St Mary's, would do his best to get a reprieve for her if he was asked. Mrs Stott said there was no chance of a reprieve: she must prepare for her doom. After this remark it was some time before Mary Ann could speak calmly. She kept touching and adjusting her hair throughout most of the visit which lasted some two hours, and she cried again when Mrs Stott rose to leave.

Mrs Stott's grand-daughter, living not far from South Hetton, told me her family spoke of Mary Ann as being clean and often kind and they thought that very probably she had not poisoned as often as people said, although the *Newcastle Journal* of the day reported that in Mrs Stott's opinion Mary Ann's wicked habits tended to shorten her mother's life. There was a report that there were other visitors that day, and that relatives of William Mowbray, two at least, were not allowed in.

The same day she wrote to James Robinson, her surviving husband.

March the 12

my dear frend
I so pose you Will mor then I can tell you conserning my Afull faite i have come I Wish to know if you will Let me see the 3 Childer as soune as you posible you can I should Like to see you Bring them if you can not Aske sum Won Eals to Bring them i have been told today you say you onley had Won Letter from me since i left you if you have not got Enny mor they have been detaining from you ie hope you Will get this And i thinke if you have Won sarke of kindness in you Will Try to get my Life spared you know your sealfe there has been A moast dredfull to hear tell of the Lyies that has been told A Bout me ie must tell you you Ar th Cause of All my trouble fore if you had not Left th house And So As i could hav got in to my house When i came the dor i Was to Wandr the steets With my Baby in my Armes no home fore me no place to Lay my head you Know if you call your mind Backe i should not solde my things in susicke street to come to you then i had mother to call on then But When you closed the dore i had no Won for you Know your sealfe i Am Knot guilty of the Lyies that has been tolde Consirnig me if you speake the nothing .But the trouth i can not draw my mind on the past for it is mor then natur can bare Won thing i hope you Will try to get my Life spared for ie Am not guilty of the crime ie have to dyie fore considr things And do What you Can fore me so ie must Conclude At this time i hope to hear from you By return of post

yor K W

M A R
M A Cotton

How odd to ask to see the children – one of them hers – even without Robinson coming with them. An aggressive letter – 'if you have one spark of kindness in you . . . you are the cause of all my trouble.' No reference to her own behaviour which lost Robinson's trust. Of course she was right about that crucial locked door. If Robinson had been at home in Pallion, a humble Mary Ann, with some time elapsed, might have rewon some sympathy: the rough time she was having would have ended and there would have been no Cotton family and West Auckland in her life. There's the past, a raw wound she could not bear to look at: to Holdforth she said it was too heartrending to think about, and to Robinson she could not think about it. 'M A R' at the end will be Mary Ann Robinson, but what is, 'K W'? Something wife?

Robinson did not reply and Mary Ann wrote to him again on the Friday, 14th March, a letter revealing growing agitation about nothing being done on her behalf and the painful knowledge that much more could have been done for her in the courts.

My de frend As i
Can not say Enny thing Ealse to you my Last request is to you Will you meeat Ant hulbard tomorrow After now forn 3 to 4 in the Afternoone you Will meeat hir beside the Banke yon side of the Bridge MunkWormouth she Wans Wans to see you ie have Wrote to try to get A portichion to get my Life spored And to come out And Stand the tryill for the othr 3 casess thot i ame carged With for ie Am not not guilty of them my proper Evidens Was not propley given to the Counsleur ie should not been condemd to death i ingaeged A man they Call him Smith i thate he Wis i solisete At frist Whun he come to me he got A bout £20 bloing to me for my first case he tolde me on the day i Was tryied At Auklang ie Was not to Speake A Single Worde And that mr Blackwell And greenhow Would be thare to defende mee When ie Went in to the docke thore Was nowon for me the Jugdge A pointed the Counsler ie must say he Was A clever man to for if he had My propr defence i should Won th tryile so i hope you Will meat hir my Lost requet

farewell
form M A R or M A Cotton

The Greenhow she mentioned was in fact one of Russell's prosecution team. Robinson did not go to meet the relation, Aunt Hulbard, Mary Ann's mother's sister: his excuse was that there was a misunderstanding about the day, and evidently he did not seek her out afterwards. He did come to the prison, however, on the Sunday, with his brother-in-law, a shopkeeper called Burns, of Prospect Row, Sunderland, and showing Mary Ann's letters asked that Burns be allowed in in his stead.

Burns was surprised to find her in a fairly big and comfortable room, although it was sparsely furnished. There were two religious books on the table. While he was there the two attendant wardresses sat on the bed while another nursed the baby. Mary Ann was dismayed not to see Robinson, and no doubt to hear the conveyed remark that he did not intend to have himself disturbed by seeing her. She asked about the children, and who was looking after them, and then urged Burns to get up a petition for her. More forcibly than Mrs Stott, Burns implored her to make her peace with God, and if she were guilty, to confess. Mary Ann said she was not guilty of poisoning Charles Edward.

'But suppose you are guilty of only one of the charges, it's the same, it's murder,' Burns said.

'But I never gave poison to anybody I know of,' she said. 'I am only guilty of bigamy, and of having this child.'

The prison chaplain, the Revd J. C. Lowe, also exhorted her to confess, but at this time the promotion of a successful petition was her dominating thought. No relative or close acquaintance, no one from the old days at South Hetton, petitioned for a reprieve – the *Northern Echo* said this showed the good moral tone of the community; but petitions, more powerful than any relative could have organized, were being thought about in Sunderland and Darlington.

On Tuesday, the 18th, the Sunderland Quaker, Edward Backhouse, sent a memorial to the Secretary of State from people who had known or employed Mary Ann in Sunderland. Edward Allan Maling, now surgeon to Sunderland Infirmary; the secretary to the infirmary; the surgeon to the Smyrna House Home for Fallen Women, and the matron, assistant matron and laundress were the memorialists, in addition to Backhouse and his wife and two others, one of them Agnes Place, who with her husband ran a pawnbroker's shop at the Borough Road corner of Sussex Street.

To the minute to him, 'Former employers of this prisoner memorialise for commutation of capital sentence on the ground that her crime was not absolutely proved,' the Home Secretary, Mr Bruce, noted, 'Nil. Ack.'

On the same day a Darlington solicitor, John T. Nixon, forwarded a petition to the Queen asking for commutation. 130 people in Darlington and Barnard Castle signed it. Among the descriptions were doctor of medicine, chemist, Primitive Methodist minister, miner, labourer, weaver, dyer, miller, cooper, brewer, seedsman, flax dresser, bank manager, innkeeper, boot-maker, gunmaker, whitesmith, blacksmith, wheelwright, and following each other L. Delmar O'Reilly, gentleman, and Bernard O'Reilly, rag merchant.

Nixon wrote that the result of this most extraordinary and important case could spread a feeling of insecurity and alarm. There had been adverse comments in part of the local press for months before the trial: the enquiry before the magistrates was removed to the eve of the trial, and so excitement was at its height when the trial was held. The verdict was purely of circumstantial evidence on an assumption of cruelty not borne out by the evidence – on the contrary, disproved by it. The assumption of hypocrisy appeared to be gratuitous, and although the law dispensed with proof of motive the mind asked for it, and one could look in vain for it. Being but a stepmother Mary Ann was under no obligation to maintain the child, a fact which appeared to escape attention. That the boy survived her own child raised doubts about her guilt.

Because of her penury she could not call upon an expert of equal or greater experience and standing to Dr Scattergood, whose conclusions were accepted unchallenged, except by Dr Richardson who, it is understood, maintained that Nattrass died of the illness entered on the certificate. The observations and opinions of the several medical attendants were put aside as valueless before the testimony of one scientific man. The absence of symptoms peculiar to arsenical poisoning did not prevent a sweeping conclusion that each had died of such poisoning. The assumption of such poisoning from the absence of other diseases, and the observation of inflammatory action after the bodies had been buried for so long, appeared to be very questionable and dangerous. Dr Scattergood's opinion of an important point had been questioned by the *Lancet* of 15th March. Dr Kilburn and his assistant contradicted each other as to whether arsenic in powder was on the shelf: Kilburn denied he had any; Chalmers said there was some there. This was so material a fact that the defence counsel wrote to the press about it.

Medicine bottles in Mary Ann's house should have been analysed. Sergeant Hutchinson said they were empty and he thought Dr Kilburn took some of them. The doctor said he did not take any. This was a very material discrepancy: knowledge of what had been in the bottles was an essential link missing in a case depending on circumstantial evidence.

It was not authorized by any law, human or divine, to imperil the tender and innocent life of a child born in prison and suckled there by its mother, by the destruction of the mother.

The Home Office minute says: 'to spare this woman's life inasmuch as the evidence against her, did not, in their opinion, satisfactorily disprove that the crime imputed to her was not the result of pure accident: they urge that the prisoner's kindly disposition bears out such a view and that her life should not be sacrificed without further consideration.'

The *Lancet* had said they did not agree with Scattergood's statement that fine particles of arsenic floating in the air could not get into a person's stomach. Arsenic had a specific irritating effect on the mucous membranes of the alimentary tract, no matter in what way it entered the system. There were remote inflammatory effects due to the absorption of the poison into the blood. Inflammatory changes in the stomach had been observed after inhalation, or the application of arsenic to a wound. If solid particles were inhaled through the mouth and nose many would adhere to membranes and find their way to the stomach.

The *Lancet* said the most interesting point of the case was perhaps the very small amount of direct evidence against Mary Ann. Had her history been less suspicious it was possible that the jury might not have been so easily satisfied. As it was, however, there could be no doubt that the verdict and sentence were just. The theories put forward by the defence had been interesting but untenable. That a mistake in the prescription had been made had no effect upon the jury. That a fine powder of arsenic had found its way into the system of the child could not be supported, as the prisoner herself had shown no symptoms of poisoning, and also too much arsenic had been found in the child to be accounted for in this manner.

The journal ended by saying that to determine between chronic arsenic poisoning and typhoid fever was no easy matter.

To John Nixon's petition the Home Secretary added his initials: 'Nil. HAB.'

Also on the 18th Martha Olive, of Grove Cottage, Dorchester, wrote to the Home Secretary,

> I have just heard with the most extreme horror that the poor woman Cotton is to be executed on Monday next. Can it be really possible that there can be a law that would take the life of a mother who has a sucking child? It is too horrible to conceive. Surely this must be a great sin before the Lord.

> I dare say that in a state of ? she thought the child would be better off than she could do for it. It appears she was very kind to all she knew, and was always ready to do a kind act.
>
> I do pray, humbly pray, that her life may be spared, and that the Lord may incline your heart to order a reprieve.

The Home Secretary's note is 'Nil. Ack.'

Henry Austin Bruce, the Home Secretary, shared an achievment with Mary Ann, although neither would be aware of it. Each was the parent of twelve children. Eight of Bruce's children were to his second wife, the daughter of the historian, Sir William Napier. Other than that, in being married more than once, and in living on the same island at the same time, the two would have little in common. Bruce, a Welshman, entered the chambers of an uncle, a lord-justice, and he was called to the bar when only twenty-two. Six years later, in 1843, he came into a fortune. In 1873 he was raised to the peerage, and became the first Baron Aberdare, Lord President of the Council. Gladstone regarded him as 'a heaven-sent Home Secretary.' He was 'a convinced member of the Church of England and the most clubable of men'.

On Wednesday, 19th March, a traumatic day for Mary Ann when her child was taken from her, forcibly, another memorial was sent from Sunderland, this time from more than 160 leading citizens including four justices of peace, the recent Under Sheriff of the county, Alderman Ranson, and the editor of the *Sunderland Times*. Forwarding the petition, A. W. Common, J. P. said the memorialists humbly prayed that the extreme penalty of the law be not carried out. The next day Common sent twenty-three more signatures. The Home Secretary initialled his 'Nil.'

Edward Backhouse wrote to William Tallack at the Home Office:

> Couldst thou see Mr Bruce and represent to him the contents of the enclosed paper, drawn up by George Smith Ranson, late Under Sheriff for the County of Durham, Attorney at Law. He proposed and I encouraged it.
>
> I sent up a Memorial yesterday for those who formerly knew or employed Mary Ann Cotton. She was once in our employ: she was recommended to me by E. Allan Maling, surgeon to the Sunderland Infirmary, as an active clever

person who had been a nurse, under him, in the Sunderland Infirmary fever ward.

All these memorials ask that the extreme penalty be not carried out as the evidence is but presumptive or circumstantial.

Canst thou do what is in thy power to represent these things.

Mr Ranson was present at the Trial.

Very truly, thy friend,
Edward Backhouse.

Backhouse added: 'Now that public opinion is cooler I have met with many who do not think her guilt proven; indeed I have not met with one who asserts it is entirely proved.'

Writing to Backhouse, Ranson said that Tallack should urge that if Mary Ann had been tried at the winter assizes she would have been acquitted as there was no other charge against her then.

On Friday, 21st March, after midday, as Mary Ann's last weekend approached, Backhouse telegraphed the Home Secretary at Whitehall – Bruce was in Bangor at the time. Backhouse said that in order to prove that evidence was admitted on other charges on which Mary Ann was not tried he would send six newspapers by fast post. Charles Russell, he said, doubted such admissibility himself: this would probably appear in the judge's notes.

The Society of Friends in Sunderland, among them wealthy merchants, also sent a memorial of 49 signatures. 116 people signed another petition from Robert Green, gentleman, of Albert Hill, near Darlington. They included many women describing themselves as 'lady'. Green pleaded that the extreme penalty should not be carried out: mistakes had sometimes occurred and innocence had been proved afterwards.

Also on the 20th an impressively argued plea was sent to Bruce by a Sunderland architect, Frank Caws. He said, But for her poverty Mary Ann could have called on homeopathic doctors to prove that gastric fever and arsenical poisoning might be the same thing – that the fever might have left arsenical deposits: that arsenic was administered as a curative for gastric fever; that some ignorant people used it occasionally as a medicine. After seeing its frequent use in the infirmary Mary Ann might have administered it, thinking it had more healing qualities than it had, not realizing the power of the poison. She had failed to see the mischief in arsenic, just as had doctors in blood-letting, in administering mercury, in repeating wrong treatment until their patients died. The prosecution had merely surmised the possession of arsenic. Unless she was insane the inducements to commit murder were insufficient. She lost more money in many of the cases than she gained.

Caws said no expense was spared by the prosecution in bringing forward witnesses. He understood that the prosecution had been asked to bring forward all their charges so that there might be time to prepare her defence, but this had not been done. The further charges were not gone into until the hearings shortly before the assizes. She had not had money to retain counsel or obtain any witnesses, scientific or otherwise, nor had she an attorney to instruct counsel to get up points in her favour.

The thirty memorialists of Sunderland and district included two solicitors and two chemists.

On the 21st the *Sunderland Times* said that efforts of the friends of humanity to have the sentence committed to life imprisonment were continuing with zeal. They believed there was a growing feeling of concern about the extraneous evidence admitted: such evidence was quite inadmissible in cases of felony or other crimes which were not capital.

The *Newcastle Daily Chronicle,* too, protested about the admitted evidence. What was the use of a specific accusation at all, except to confine evidence? The cases should have been tried separately. It was very doubtful if the 'hapless wretch' had fair trial.

A letter to the paper supported Mr Justice Archibald. W. W. Robson of Sunderland, outlining the case of Mary Ann Geering, said even if Mrs Cotton's counsel had not indicated an intention of setting up a theory of accidental poisoning, surely the prosecution was entitled to show that death was not accidental.

On that Friday an urgent telegraph from the Home Office came to Colonel Armstrong. Did thoughts that this was a reprieve streak through his mind? The telegraph followed one from the Home Secretary to his office.

> From H. A. Bruce, The Palace, Bangor.
> To Hon. A Liddell, Home Office, London.
> Please ascertain through Governor of
> prison whether there is any
> truth in the statement that
> Mary Ann Cotton is pregnant.

The telegraph, five words to a line for threepence, cost a shilling. It was handed in at 10.33 in the morning and sent out at 11.20. Liddell must have moved fast, as Armstrong's reply to the Home Office, costing one and threepence, was handed in at Durham at 1.33 p.m. Armstrong said,

> It is *not* true that
> Mary Ann Cotton is pregnant
> She had a child born
> in prison on the seventh
> of January letter by post.

His letter, written that day, says,

> It is *utterly untrue* that Mary Ann Cotton is pregnant. She was committed on 23rd August last, being then with child, and would have been tried at the Assizes held here on the 10th December but for her state of health. She was confined of a female child on the 7th January, which child was given over to some friends of hers to be brought up, the day before yesterday, the 19th, it being then in good health.

The earnest, pleading Quaker, Edward Backhouse, posted his six newspapers to Bruce that day. He said that without the extraneous evidence there would not have been a conviction, adding a doubting, weakening 'probably.' Bruce instructed, 'nil.'

CHAPTER SEVEN

The hanging

Hoping We Will All Meeat in heaven
at gods Write hand.

In her room Mary Ann gradually, eventually faced the seeming certainty that her life was going to be deliberately terminated by the working-out of the law: that she was going to be killed as punishment, as an act of social justice, for what others had agreed that she had done.

She was in a special, an extraordinary position. She had times when she was lost in thought, sometimes she was obviously in a depression. These times often ended with an outburst of protesting or by her being overwhelmed with grief. She would recover, be silent, apart again, seemingly calm, even occasionally indifferent: then there would be the slip into waiting despair. She would speak aloud to God, praying from her bed, from her chair, suddenly speaking out, beseeching solace, understanding, guidance, and also asking for the protection of her child. During the night her guardians would notice her watching them, her eyes flashing in the firelight.

Five days before the day set for the execution the baby girl was taken from her and the cradle was suddenly missing from the room. She had spoken of the father taking the child but the excise man just wanted to keep out of things. She had wondered if the child would have to go into the workhouse at Bishop Auckland, but, in fact, there were many people willing to take the baby and adopt it, some of them well-to-do. It was said there were a hundred and fifty applicants, one of them a Bishop Auckland J.P. There was surprised comment in the press when Mary Ann chose foster-parents in humble circumstances: Sarah and William Edwards of Johnson Terrace. The couple, twenty-nine-years-old, were childless after seven years of marriage. Edwards, a Welshman, was a miner at St Helen's Auckland Colliery.

Early in that last week rumours got outside that she had intended to make the child ill in the hope of delaying the execution. A small piece of soap was missing in her room. Soap was occasionally swallowed by prisoners: it had a purging effect and could cause a low fever. It was a device resorted to after the introduction of the treadmill and partly accounted for the increase in illness in prisons. Mary Ann maintained she knew nothing about the soap, but the piece was found up her sleeve.

On Wednesday, 19th March, the Edwardses and William Lowrey, Mary Ann's last lodger, came for the baby. That evening Lowrey wrote about his day to the *Northern Echo*.

> I got a letter from Mrs Cotton last week asking me to try and get up a petition to save her life. I sent word back that I thought there would be no chance for her and told her, in my simple way, to come to the cross of Christ, for He says, 'Let your sins be as red as scarlet, I will make them as white as snow. He that cometh unto me I will in no way cast out.' When I was writing Mr and Mrs Edwards told me to ask her if she would give them the baby, and they would assure her that they would bring it up in the fear of God.
>
> I got a letter last night. It came by train, and the St Helen's station master brought it down. Many thanks for his kindness. She was quite willing for Mr Edwards to have the baby, and very thankful in him besides for his kindness. So we were up by the lark this morning, and arrived at the prison by 9.30 a.m. We had a bit of trouble getting in, but thanks to Mr Fawcett, he gave an order for our admission. So, after leaving our watches and little property at the office inside the door, we were taken to the cell where the unhappy woman was. I found the cell fifty times better than I expected. Everything was as clean as a new pin. The first thing I saw was Mrs Cotton sitting on a stool close to a good fire, giving the breast to her infant. She was dressed in a skirt, a loose jacket, but no shoes on, and nothing on her head. Looking round the cell I saw three chairs, one table, a bed and some good books. The walls had pretty paper on. There was one window on the south side and the sun was shining on it. In fact she seems to have every comfort that this earth can afford. God forbid, Mr Editor, that I should ever see such a sight again. Just imagine a little child on its mother's knee, looking up at its mother's

face and laughing, and her on the brink of another world, and her heart as hard as a stone. These are the words she said:

'I wish I may never have any power to rise off this seat. I never gave that boy Charles Edward any poison wilfully. It was in the arrowroot, and all got it. I am going to die for a crime I am not guilty of.'

But nevertheless we got the child home all right. It has a kind father and mother: may God bless them. I may just say that the female warders are very kind to her.

Mrs Edwards told a *Northern Echo* reporter later that she was allowed in when she showed the letter from Mary Ann but the two men had to seek out a magistrate in the city for permission. Mary Ann cut her black and white shawl in halves and wrapped a half round the baby. She said to her: 'Promise me that you'll never let Riley come near where it is; never, never. And promise me if it should be bad, that you'll never have Dr Kilburn attend it.' She made these promises. Since then Riley had called at her house, and she had had to ask him to go away.

Mary Ann's statement about the arrowroot – which she was to repeat – was as far as she went towards admitting responsibility. She was saying that the shopkeeper who sold the arrowroot, through carelessness probably, had mixed arsenic with it. It looks pretty certain that she said she bought the arrowroot at Riley's shop, as the *Northern Echo* reporter went to the shop and asked about this. Riley's son said Mary Ann could have bought the arrowroot there. He said she had certainly bought soothing syrup there. Her credit had been stopped at the shop when it reached thirty shillings.

The taking away of the child must have seemed the start of the end. The child had been new life to feel and see, close to her, fed by her. She could well have had illusory thoughts that no one would really have the baby taken from her and then have her led to the scaffold. She held on to the child and the forced separation distressed everyone in the room.

Mary Ann could not respond to the words of the chaplain, the Revd J. C. Lowe, and on the Thursday when two visiting justices came to see her, the Revd A. D. Shafto and Mr Rowland Burdon, she confided to each in turn that she would like to see a Wesleyan minister. The result was that the Revd W.

Stevenson, of the Durham Wesleyan Circuit, was summoned to the prison. There was sympathetic communication immediately: he brought back thoughts and feelings of her youth when she went to chapel and Sunday school, and he softened the aspect of her short, grim future. When, on his leaving, the attendants returned to the room, she told them she was happier than she had been. Stevenson left her a hymn book and this she carried about, sometimes reading aloud from it with such comments as, 'Isn't that beautiful?'

It was well she was finding solace. It had been decided that the place of execution would be the same as that for the last hangings – of two Spennymoor brothers-in-law, just over two months before. The men, Hugh Slane and John Hays, had been found guilty of kicking a man to death. The cavity for the drop had been left, on the eastern side of the prison near to the shot-drill ground. The warrant of execution had been received by the Sheriff and the black gallows, used for Slane and Hays, was being erected. William Calcraft, last public hangman, was due to leave his home in Hoxton to come north. He had been coming to Durham as 'finisher of the law,' since 1865 when the previous hangman's rope had snapped. Calcraft persisted in using the 'short drop,' being concerned at the possibility of the head being wrenched off by the 'long drop.' This was to happen twelve years later at Norwich. Calcraft's victims often lived a few convulsive minutes and sometimes he would go into the pit and pull at the body with all his weight – 'to steady their legs a little,' was a euphemism of his. In evidence before the Commission on Capital Punishment in 1864 it was said that Calcraft's method of hanging was very rough, rather as if he were hanging a dog. William Marwood, who followed Calcraft as the main executioner, used the 'long drop'. He said Calcraft hanged people; he himself executed them.

Although Calcraft had performed many public hangings, including the last one, at Newgate, in May, 1868, he had resented the press being allowed in the pinioning-room at Durham when he had strapped Hays and then Slane. Because of this, the visiting justices that Thursday resolved that the reporters would not see Mary Ann strapped and that only one representative of a newspaper office would be allowed to witness the hanging. It was thought then – before the advent of the Wesleyan minister – that Mary Ann could well struggle in an attempt to stop her arms being pinioned, and that she would refuse to make the walk to the scaffold and would have to be conveyed there strapped in a chair and be hanged from this sitting position. Maybe it was because of this fear that Calcraft was to have an assistant.

A chair had been used in one of his worst hangings, that of William Bousfield at Newgate. Bousfield had tried to burn himself in his cell and appeared to be so weak that four men carried him to the scaffold and he was put in a chair there. When the drop was operated, after hanging for some seconds, he raised himself and actually got his feet to the top of the cavity. He was pushed off and swung by his neck, but managed again to get a foot on the top. When he was pushed off for the fourth time, Calcraft got into the cavity himself and clung round Bousfield's middle, tugging until he was strangled.

On the Friday Stevenson visited Mary Ann three times. She knew of the petitions, certainly of the one from the Society of Friends, but Stevenson seems to have realized there was very little hope and to have conveyed this. Most of her time she read or looked at religious books.

On the Saturday morning she was pleased when a letter arrived from William Edwards telling her how the baby was and of the many people who had called in to see it:

West Auckland.
March 20/73.

My Dear friend
how are you by this time I think it is my Duty to write you a few lines and let you know how your little Baby is getting on. Wee arrive home all right. Wee had many hundreds of visiters to see it and they say it is a fine one. amongst them we had Mr and Mrs Maughan and there Daughter. Poor Little thing it had a pretty good night. But a better day. but you must not let It trouble your mind for it will be all right by Gods Help. I may just say Mrs Edward hopes wee will all meet in a better world we Remain your Most Respectfull
William and Sarah Edwards.

Lowrey added a note on the back page of the good-quality four-page notepaper which could well have distressed, especially with the self-indulgent emotionalism of its ending, 'goodby on this Earth *for ever*.'

Mrs Cotton it ote to be a great comfort to you to think that the Lord has been so kind to you to have porvieded a kind Father and Mother for your Child. for *Lord* sacke put your whole trust in the lord *Juses* Christ for he says She that will Confess there sins I will forgive them Just look at it in another world never never no end May the lord have Mercy on your Soul goodby on this Earth *for ever*
Lowrey.

Mary Ann showed the letter from the Edwards to her attendants. It is one of a number fortunately retained by the prison matron, Margaret Robinson, and held by a relation.

She wrote two short last letters that day – both delivered the next day, Sunday: the one to Lowrey about Smith and the pawn tickets given in Chapter Two, and a reply to the Edwards:

My dear frends

I reseved yours this morning And happy to hear my Baby was well I hope by the healpe of god she Will grow in grase And repay you for your kindness to her I hope she Will be a blessing to you Both so you must Excuse my shorte note to you As ie feale unable to Write more hoping We Will All Meeat in heaven at gods Write hand Where ther Will be no more pain

Yours Affnelnedly
Mary Ann Cotton

March th 22, 1873
Kiss my Babe for me.

There is acceptance there: the good influence of Stevenson is evident. The child did grow in grace . . . in tribulation certainly, as will be seen. As for the other note one would think that Lowrey, inconsiderately, had grumbled to her about not being able to get the clothes out of pawn and her letting them go to Smith. The letters from prison prompted the *Northern Echo* to say, 'We do not envy the heart of him who has read unmoved the letters from the condemned cell. Letters more touching, more horribly pathetic we have seldom seen. The rude, inarticulate manner in which they are expressed, their earnest, their terrible earnest pleading for life, and the desperate manner in which they attack everyone and grasp at anything, render them more painful than anything we have seen for years.'

She would also receive that day, or on the Sunday, the following letter, of growing fervour, from an old friend in South Hetton, Matthew Hall:

South Hetton Mar 21st – 1873

My Dear unfortunate Friend, I embrace the only opportunity that may now be left me, of giving unto you the only Counsel that may be of Service in your Awful position, apparently to all human knowledge, so near your Doom. I have just read your Letter to Holdforth, in the Daily Paper and you appear to have cast your thoughts back on your former days, when a Sabbath School Teacher, when your Dear Mother was also a Member of the Wesleyan Society, these were Happy days – and you know it – you had a good Mother and a good bringing up. You were taught the Principles of the Religion of the Bible and now where are you. As one that Loves your Soul, I do not here upbraid you of anything that you may have done, that is known best by yourself, and most assuredly by God, but I earnestly entreat you to make good use of the short time, that, to all appearance, you have to live. You seem to have a Hope of Heaven – be sure that Hope is well founded. A mere formal notion, or wish, will avail you nothing, you must seek it earnestly with your whole heart, and with Tears – let not a moment slip – banish the idea of a Reprieve from your mind so long as you hang upon this notion, your Heart and Soul will not be fully in earnest – Life is sweet, but you cannot rely upon this uncertainty – But you can place your implicit Confidence upon Christ's Atonement – This my Dear Mary Ann is the important Duty you must perform – and without delay – Heaven is a Happy Place – but none go there unpardoned and unholy – that great change must be effected here on Earth. I charge you therefore as I write in the presence of God to take heed and let not your Soul be be Lost through negligence or delay – but make immediate Effort and seek the Saviour – may God help you is my earnest prayer – and now my Dear Unfortunate friend I take my leave of you to all appearance upon Earth – and I trust you take the advice your best of friends give unto you – so God Bless you and Farewell.

Matthew Hall
South Hetton.

To Mary Ann Cotton
Inmate of Durham Jail.

Probably as good a letter as she could receive in the circumstances, although it would have been better if the statements about her imminent doom had been omitted.

There was more of this to be endured from her last visitor from outside, other than the Wesleyan ministers. This was her stepfather, George Stott, then a deputy overman at Seaham Colliery, a man, said the *Durham County Advertiser*, of a 'religious turn of mind'. The visit was too late to be of any material help and it is very doubtful if solace was gained from it. Mary Ann, gazing into the fire, jumped up when Stott appeared and hugging him said she knew he would come and see her. Stott impressed upon her the gravity of her position; he told her – wrongly – the petitions had not been forwarded to the Home Office; he said he was surprised at her bad spelling, shown in her letters printed in the newspapers, and that she must have lost the education she received in early life. Mary Ann observed it was no matter of wonder that she spelt badly and wrote badly (which she didn't) considering the position she was in and what she had to think of.

She told her stepfather she was innocent, but that she might have been instrumental in causing the death of Charles Edward. But not by intention, she said. She had bought arrowroot from a grocer in West Auckland and he had made up the quantity with something else of a different colour from another drawer and it was this which had poisoned the boy. The explanation, understandably, did not impress Stott, who felt he was the only person she was likely to confess to. There was a sufficiency of shared and known life between them to cause them to weep together. She had to be consoled when he left. She asked him if he would see Robinson for her.

Shortly before five that day, Saturday, the 22nd, William Calcraft got off the London express at Durham station. In him the personification of death was a small, stooped, dark-suited man of seventy-three with a bearded and wrinkled face. He walked unsteadily. He had begun at Newgate in his middle twenties, flogging children for ten shillings a week. He had been hanging people for a very long time, for some forty-five years, since before Victoria was Queen. He did not know how many people he had hanged. One or two of his grandchildren usually accompanied him when he went to collect his guinea a week retainer in London. He received a guinea extra for each hanging and half-a-crown for each flogging. For trips into the country such as this he was usually paid £10. Such was his standing that the hanging of three men in January had been postponed. Slane and Hays at Durham and a man at Liverpool were all due to be executed on 6th January. Calcraft arrived at Liverpool thinking that the Durham hangings had been postponed for a week when he would be available, only to find it was the Liverpool hanging which had been postponed. His final hanging was fourteen months ahead, and afterwards the city of London granted him a pension of 25s. a week. He liked pigeons and pet animals. The *Newcastle Chronicle*, on that visit, spoke of the infamy of the man and his judicial murders.

Calcraft went straight to the gaol where he had been given quarters, and either in the short time before darkness that evening or on the Sunday morning, he looked at the pit under the gallows and said it would have to be widened and deepened to take a chair.

His assistant, Robert Evens, who could well have travelled north with him, was a few years younger, a fairly prosperous Welshman in his sixties who had his own farm near Carmarthen. He was a tall, lithe, strongly-built man of quick movements. Although he had been a hangman for fourteen years he did not want his name known and there was a deal of speculation about it for a day or so. It was said that at his farm he had his hanging-rope hung up in the sitting-room. He stayed close to the prison, at the Court Inn nearby.

Mary Ann would probably be unaware of the hangmen's arrival and it is doubtful if she was concerned about how far she would drop when the floor fell away from her. One imagines she expected an instantaneous leaving of this world for another. Two more Wesleyan ministers had been to see her, the Revd J. M. Mountford, superintendent of the Durham circuit, and the Revd J. Bennett. The Revd Lowe had told her that he would be with her on her final walk. That night she fell asleep in her chair reading the Bible. 'Let me alone for a while,' she complained when she was wakened, but shortly afterwards she went to bed.

On Sunday morning Bennett was round to see her at six and he stayed for two hours. She had a spell of euphoria saying that she was happy and that she was prepared to die; that her Saviour had had a bitter death and had been spat upon: she would not be spat upon and He would be with her and would make her passing peaceful. Soon, she said to her warders, she would meet her mother and father in heaven. Later she had a recurrence of wishing her relatives and friends had done more for her; that her defence had been better at the outset; and that witnesses had been called to give evidence in her favour. She repeated to Bennett that she was innocent so forcibly that although he could not believe her, he was impressed and disturbed.

In the prison chapel and in local churches prayers were offered up for her: at the Wesleyan chapel in Durham, at the parish church of St Oswald's, and in the afternoon at Durham cathedral. In his sermon there the Bishop of Dover said that she for whom they had especially prayed was in more than an ordinary sense under sentence of death: it was not impossible that forgiveness might even be extended to her.

There was a fair amount of sympathy for her now. The baby taken from her so that she could be killed; the helplessness of her position; a fading of revulsion and of the certainty of her guilt; the knowledge of her fervent return to the Wesleyan faith made some feel she would not really be executed; others accepted what was to happen with sorrow.

On Sunday afternoon Stevenson was with her for nearly two hours, and he began to have doubts that she had poisoned anyone intentionally; he began to feel that she was not guilty of wilful murder. When first summoned he had been convinced of her guilt. He returned again that evening. She was reading the hymns, keeping herself close to the only thoughts and wording which could bring her comfort. She held on to the assurance that dying was only a bridge, that soon she would be with people she had known, with them in peace and love. She asked Stevenson if he would write letters of thanks for her, particularly to the Edwards. He left promising to be back at six in the morning.

She went to bed about half-past ten. For a long time she was restless, moaning occasionally, and then for some three hours her watchers thought she had a deeper rest. She was wide awake about four in the morning and soon got up. They helped her to dress. She could not face a breakfast but had a cup of tea at half-past five. Before six the three Wesleyan ministers arrived. She was fervent in prayer and asked that the female warders be brought back into the room so that they could join in the prayers, and she prayed for them. She mentioned especially her last baby, her last legal husband, Robinson, and her stepfather.

Mountford broached the advisability of a confession. What she said in response, whatever it was, was not the same as she had told him before, and he spoke to her about this. Later, he said she had been the agent, the means; she had been the poisoner, but not intentionally. He said to her, 'You know, Mrs Cotton, it is not one act, done upon one day, and embracing one case. Months passed over and those persons of your family died. You admit that you have done it, but, you say, not intentionally. How did those deaths occur in that way?' But there was no more from her. That morning, upset before the pressmen, he said he had hoped and thought that something more was coming from her, he had urged her to say more, but there had been no more. There was no open confession. Those who knew her best had not expected any.

One of the shocking surprises which living still held for Mary Ann was the sight of those who had come to watch her put to death. The reporters, some two dozen of them, began to assemble outside the gates soon after seven. It was a damp, misty morning. Other people were drawn there to wait for the fateful hour, to see the black flag run up, and perhaps to hear the releasing platform doors crash open. Calcraft must have moved to the Court Inn or gone there early that morning because the reporters saw both hangmen walking towards them. One reporter described their walk as sauntering. Evens was wearing a shiny broad-brimmed hat. The reporters stood aside for the two men and Calcraft gave them a grin. In the comments among themselves which followed the reporters who didn't know were told of the identity of Evens.

Shortly afterwards, on presentation of their passes, the pressmen filed into the prison and were taken to stand under some roof-covering. It was as if there was nothing happening: deserted scene, the odd noise muted. Then Calcraft and Evens walked across the yard at pace, making for the female quarters. The pressmen knew they had gone to do the pinioning. Then quietness and stillness returned.

One would expect that the reporters would remember the last of Slane and Hays just over two months before. They had seen Calcraft enter the pinioning-room carrying his straps. Hays, cap in hand, had wanted to address them, but the officials, anxious to have the dreadful task finished with, assured him that his written statement about his innocence would be shown to them – as indeed it was. Hays had had to be content with that. He stood, a thick woollen comforter round his neck, face to face with Calcraft. The hangman unwound the scarf and bared Hays's neck. Slane, watching, took off his own scarf. Calcraft put a broad leather belt round Hays, pinioning his arms but leaving his hands holding his cap. He then did the same to Slane.

And then there was the scene at the gallows: ropes dangling in the breeze; Calcraft waiting at the furthest side of the platform, and then, when the procession had reached him, so busy, attempting to crack jokes with the officials, grinning, all in front of the two men. After strapping their legs, he had shaken hands with them. And when it was all over and the two lifeless figures swayed slowly, the hands of Hays still grasped the cap the late living man had taken off in the presence of his betters.

Two men that day: that was exceptional – although Calcraft had also hanged two men at Durham in 1869 on his previous visit – and now a woman, also exceptional. After Mary Ann's sentence some of the reporters had written about that last execution of a woman at Durham, that of Mary Nicholson in 1799. The rope had snapped and before another could be got Mary Nicholson recovered and talked with her relatives. She had to wait nearly an hour for a new rope to be brought. Mary had waited to be sentenced too, for nearly a year after being found guilty of causing the death of her mistress by putting poison in a pudding. During that time she had been a servant in the prison, sometimes being sent into the city on errands on her own.

But, at a quarter to eight on that morning of 24th March, 1873, the reporters dismissed any retrospective thoughts they might have had as they were led to wait in the Governor's office. The office looked out between the south and east wings; the east wing in fact ran obliquely south-east so that the view was a limited one. Near the end of the east wing there stood the gallows. Two uprights were driven into the ground, a beam across the top. The rope with its noose hung from an iron eyebolt in the centre. The platform, at ground level over the pit, was a pair of folding doors, hinged at the outside and held horizontal by an iron frame slid underneath. This was drawn back and away by pulling it with a handle or lever or bolt.

At about ten minutes to eight the St Oswald's passing-bell tolled over the city, and the death-bell was sounded in the prison. It was heard in Mary Ann's crowded apartment. Her face was strained and pinched, her wide, fine eyes bright with tears. Could any thinking, sensitive person look her in the face? That still left a lot of people who could, of course. The feeling man, having to accept that the killing must take place, just wanted it over, so that he, and she, could be freed of this time.

Colonel Armstrong was away that harrowing morning – called to give evidence before a parliamentary committee in London considering a new gas company bill – so James Young, his deputy, was the person in the room who received the demand to hand over the body of Mary Ann Cotton. The Under Sheriff, Richard Bowser of Bishop Auckland, and his deputy, E. G. Marshall arrived outside the apartment with the bailiff, two warders and Calcraft and Evens behind them. Bowser and Marshall entered the room and made the demand.

They then stood out of the way, allowing Evens to dart in quietly. Suddenly Mary Ann's arms were grasped and held to her sides. She gasped and stood subdued while a broad and strong leather belt was strapped around her arms and chest. She clasped and unclasped her free hands. She was asked if she could walk, or if she feared this might be too much for her: would she like to be carried in a chair? She said she would walk.

The Under Sheriff's party left to wait outside the building. The reporters were brought out of the Governor's office and stationed in the men's exercise yard – the 'males' airing ground', – close to the gateway from the 'females' airing ground.' Mary Ann was led out of her apartment by the matron and by the two wardresses, Miss Robinson and Miss Jellis, who had been with her for most of the time. She said, 'Heaven is my home.' When they came through the yard door the wardresses stood back and two warders took up positions at either side, with Bennett alongside one of them. Holding her elbows, the warders led her forward. Calcraft and Evens came immediately behind, then the Deputy Governor; then Mountford, Stevenson and Lowe; then Bowser and Marshall, the bailiff, and six warders. The two wardresses followed.

The pressmen had been drawn up four deep in military fashion by Thompson Smith, the head warder, the man who had spoken for Mary Ann at Bishop Auckland against the conduct of George Smith. There was a medical student or two with them and a man called Crooks who said he was engaged on a philosophic enquiry: this had meant his presence at executions in many parts of the world.

The first indication that the procession was approaching was the sounds of the ministers praying and of Mary Ann sobbing. When the procession came through the gateway Mary Ann's head was erect, even held back a little, and she was trying to pray between her sobs. Her old black gown hung loosely on her slender frame. The half shawl had been draped round her by the wardresses to hide the strap at the front. Her head and throat were bare, her face wan and worn, her hands clasped tight together in their limited freedom. She was shivering but she walked resolutely, seeming to push herself forward, in contrast to some of those behind. She was startled to see the men in lines, her hands opened as if in amazement and her glance at them seemed to be one of almost fierce resentment. She continued to push out her feet. The gallows was not in view; it was – one imagines deliberately – just at the other side of the projecting east wing. She was three minutes away from being hanged.

The pressmen joined the procession at the back. There were only some eighty yards to walk now round the protruding building. Mary Ann's resolution began to run out: she had endured some four minutes since leaving her room. Her shivering became more noticeable as she prayed. She turned the corner of the east wing and was confronted with the gallows. She gave out an odd, strange sound – gasping, sighing and sobbing – and she leant back on to the hands and arms of the warders who hurried her forward. Calcraft and Evens slipped in front and took hold of her and she made low, unintelligible, unlistened-to ejaculations. The two wardresses could take no more: they turned away and hastened back to their quarters.

Calcraft and Evens worked quickly. They placed her on the platform, beneath the noose, turned her round so that she faced the way she had come. She was now shaking uncontrollably; her hands were clasped, and as she seemed to be saying, 'Lord, have mercy upon me. Oh, Lord, receive my soul', Evens slipped a white cap over her head, drew the noose round her neck and set the knot beneath her right ear. Calcraft strapped her ankles, tugged and checked the rope above her and as he stepped on to the side plank Evens, not waiting for a signal from the Under Sheriff, pulled the handle. The flat doors crashed open and Mary Ann dropped, her short fall ending with a jerk. Bowser, the Under Sheriff, who was supposed to drop his handkerchief as the signal, crumpled in a faint, but one or two of the warders were quick enough to stop him from falling.

Mary Ann was swinging round, her chest heaving and her

clasped hands jumping up and down. Then she began to twist about and to sway from side to side. Calcraft grasped her by the shoulder and steadied her but when he lifted his hand away she began to turn round again. Her body, unlike her mind, was loath to give up life; it waged its desperate, frightful, hopeless fight. Shocked, hurt, in pain, it writhed, threw itself, jerked, the jumping hands frustrated by the pinioned arms from easing the agony of the cap and the rope, strangling mercilessly, inefficiently.

The Times and the *Durham County Advertiser* said it was three minutes before the more or less violent movements weakened to twitchings. The *Newcastle Daily Chronicle* said Mary Ann's frame was 'terribly slow to yield the last sign of life'. There was 'an age of horror between the first convulsive spasm of the whole body and the last final shudder of the pinioned arms'. When the final twitch was over the body was left for the breezes to push and elbow, to turn at times. People moved away. The black flag had been run up at the prison gateway when the drop was heard – there were some two hundred people waiting and watching on the Court Green outside. Others had waited for the sound just over the prison wall, in the Parson's Field. The body hung for an hour after the sound. The prison surgeon then came and confirmed that Mary Ann was dead.

Calcraft untied the rope and the body was lowered on to some planks. The white cap was removed. Mary Ann's face was puffed and lurid and twisted slightly to the right. Her mouth was open, and her lips swollen. Boyd, the surgeon, said in his opinion, death had been almost instantaneous. The movements of the limbs and twitchings of the neck and breast were only muscular contortions. The body was laid in a deal coffin painted black on the outside, and taken to the prison chapel.

In London a Mr George Everest of the Home Office opened the last papers to be sent there on behalf of Mary Ann: a letter from William Tallack writing from the Howard Association in London, enclosing reports of the trial bearing out that extraneous evidence had been brought forward, and wondering if this affected the legality of the proceedings. Everest did not waste his time on a summary. His minute to the Home Secretary was: 'Recd the morning of execution.'

At ten o'clock in the morning special editions of the *Newcastle Daily Chronicle* and the *Northern Echo* were issued 'with a full account of Mrs Cotton under the drop'. At eleven the inquest on Mary Ann was held in the prison schoolroom. Mrs Stott of South Hetton, in deep mourning, accompanied by a young woman, was allowed in. She had been weeping since she came into the prison and in the schoolroom she turned her face to a wall and continued to sob. The coroner, John Favell, said his duty, 'on view of the body of Mary Ann Cotton now here lying dead at the prison at Durham,' was an unnecessary one, but the law demanded it. The jurors were taken to see Mary Ann. Gazing down at her checked shawl and black skirt one of the jurymen remarked that the rope should be with her, it should not be 'made a show of.' Favell said that he had nothing to do with the rope and neither had the juryman. Warder Appleton in charge of the body explained that the executioner was entitled to take away the rope. An argument took place over the coffin and continued in the schoolroom when they all returned there, although Mrs Stott and her companion, who had followed the jury into the chapel, remained. The juryman maintained that the rope should not be exhibited to make money. Favell said he knew of no law which said the rope must be buried with the culprit and that formerly a hangman had claimed the clothes a culprit was wearing.

The body was formally identified by the two wardresses, and Boyd, the surgeon, stated that Mary Ann died from asphyxia by hanging. In the papers sent to the Home Office it was declared that Judgment of Death was executed in the presence of the Under Sheriff; the Deputy Governor of the Gaol; the prison chaplain; George Lowlands, newspaper reporter and Joseph Moore, newspaper editor.

After the inquest two members of the West Hartlepool Phrenological Society took a cast of Mary Ann's head. The justices had granted their application to do this so that scientific knowledge could be extended. Facsimiles of the cast were to be supplied to a scientific society in Edinburgh and to Durham Gaol. To make the cast the two men cut off Mary Ann's long and shining black hair. James Young, the deputy governor, saw that all the hair, even to the last filament visible, was put back in the coffin. Lowrey had fancied himself as a phrenologist. He said of Mary Ann: 'Veneration: small. Philo-progenitiveness: almost nil. Destructiveness and secretiveness: very large. Powers of calculation: good. Language: sadly deficient.'

She was buried at two o'clock near to the west wall beside the last persons to be executed in the prison, Slane and Hays, and John Dolan and John McConville in 1869 for murders in

Sunderland and Darlington. Mrs Stott and companion attended the funeral.

The two hangmen caught the 3.05 train south. People gathered at the station to look at them. There were people waiting at Darlington station and a shout went up when Calcraft was spotted; there was a rush to the window, but the little old man with white hair leant forward and pulled the small curtains across the window.

Photographs of an impassive Mary Ann in her checked shawl were being sold by a Durham photographer. There are still a few of these about. Eight days after the hanging, on Tuesday, 1st April, an entertainment, a 'great moral drama – The Life and Death of Mary Ann Cotton', was staged at West Hartlepool's Theatre of Varieties, the New Gaiety. There were now dire tales of apparitions of lost, wailing children; of remorseless, dreadful Mary Ann. The horrific myths which obscured the shocking truth were well on their way to being formed.

CHAPTER EIGHT

A summing up

How many people did Mary Ann poison and kill? Sixteen, up to twenty or so, are the usual figures given. If she poisoned all those who died when they were dependent on her or near to her, then the number is twenty-one: her eight children by Mowbray; Mowbray himself; Ward; her mother; three of Robinson's children; the first of her children by Robinson; Cotton's sister Margaret; Cotton himself; his two boys; the baby she bore him, and Nattrass. But some of the children, the early ones especially, could well have died naturally. Perhaps fourteen or fifteen is about the truth.

There was disappointment that she did not confess, mainly to extinguish a doubt when there was no direct evidence. What an amazing state of things – no direct evidence at all, in all those deaths over the years with different doctors in attendance! That no one saw her can be accepted; but one would have thought when a search was made at the end that a trace of arsenic would have been found. However, the fact of so long remaining clear of the law is testimony of her carefulness. The *Sunderland Times*, like the *Newcastle Daily Chronicle* opposed to capital punishment, said that in almost every other civilized country positive proof was required before an execution.

There was also Christian concern over Mary Ann being killed by the State when she was impenitent. The *Sunderland Times* said, 'the law of the land, Christian society, acting on circumstantial evidence, had assumed the responsibility of her eternal damnation. If she had been imprisoned she might have become penitent before she died.' The State, the paper said, had outraged the sixth commandment: it had no right to do what the private citizen might not do: public revenge was as illegitimate as private revenge.

The *Newcastle Daily Journal*, however, spoke of her unusual nerve, cold cruelty, her heartlessness, and said no one had less title to be permitted to live. And the *Durham County Advertiser* said that the public's instinctive conviction was that the best thing for society and for Mary Ann was that she should quit the earth.

There was concern that such poisoning could have taken place without causing the doctors to be suspicious. Who was to know now what poisonings were being done? The answer was, no one. No one could know if there was no suspicion: the relatively new science of toxicology could function only after that.

Mr Justice Avory, in his charge at the trial of Jean Pierre Vaquier, said, 'Of all forms by which human nature may be overcome the most detestable is that of poison, because it can of all others be the least prevented.'

Poisoning, often arsenical, using a white, tasteless and odourless powder, had been a frightening problem for centuries. No wonder there were food-tasters; no wonder dreadful punishment was wrought on discovered poisoners. In the sixteenth century in England a statute denied poisoners benefit of clergy and said they had to be boiled.

On the Sunday before Mary Ann's execution the leader-writer of the *Northern Echo* wrote:

> We only hang our poisoners – nor do we hang all we catch. Hanging is a luxury to what might have been. Before many of our readers have opened this journal Mrs Cotton will be hanging by the neck. It is horrible. But what would it have been if Calcraft, instead of pulling a bolt and flinging apart the gates of eternity in a few seconds of time, had seized the trembling and shrieking convict, and hurled her, pinioned and helpless, into a huge cauldron in which the water was bubbling and seething with the intense heat.

The scourge of the secret poisoner can only be guessed at, particularly before the time of death certification and stricter control of the sale of poisons, and especially in England where there was a long-held-to aversion to the carrying out of autopsies. Medico-legal autopsies were held in the Italian states and in German towns centuries before medical evidence was looked to in England.

In 1838, in Mary Ann's lifetime, the first annual report of the Registrar General said that coroners and juries could not be expected to know much about poisoning as they were rarely assisted, as in other countries, by information which an examination of the body and an analysis of the stomach contents could provide. 'That poisoning,' the report says, 'may be confounded with natural disease affords a strong temptation to the criminal.'

There was nothing remarkable in the erroneous death certification. In Newcastle a survey in 1939 showed that a third of the certified causes of death were wrong, and even in 1955, when autopsies were done in over 1,400 cases in many different hospitals in Britain, nearly a fifth of the certifying physicians were wrong with their facts: nearly half wrong in their opinions. Where infants were concerned the margin of doubt was higher. It seems reasonable to say that, had other doctors attended Mary Ann's victims, they too would have seen nothing to cause them to mistrust her. The *Durham County Advertiser* asked, unnecessarily, if it was creditable to medical science that Nattrass should die with seventeen and a half grains of arsenic in him without foul play being suspected. (Richardson put down typhoid fever, as death was a bit hasty for Bright's disease.)

Those were days of the notorious burial clubs, occasionally run by undertakers. Some unfortunate children, usually girls, were entered in three or four clubs. Often children were allowed to die without any approach being made to a doctor. Throughout Mary Ann's lifetime it was common in some town districts to drug children with a mixture containing laudanum to keep them quiet. Other ingredients in the 'cordial' were aniseed and treacle. It was sold quite openly. In 1866 the coroner for Camden Town, Dr Lankester, reckoned that there were well over 400 child murders in London each year.

But did such behaviour affect Mary Ann? It is doubtful if there would be much of it about her at home in the colliery districts, where her so-young parents seem to have been thrust into a life of hard work and responsibility. There was the Wesleyan chapel and Sunday school; the letters to and from old friends in Murton and South Hetton show a Christian outlook; and there were the colliery habits of cleanliness and tidiness. And surely there was no callous behaviour in South Hetton House where there was no privation and plenty of food, activity and gay noise. But could it be that the many Potter children turned her against children? Did she there determine she would be a lady when she could, and pay others to do chores? Did the memory of the looks cast at her – a pretty nursemaid in the manager's house alongside a lively, busy pit-yard – did the memory make her grasp out for love in later years?

Life could well have become coarsened after her marriage, when she and Mowbray travelled about the south-west, and later in Sunderland, especially after Mowbray's death and before she moved in with Robinson. And perhaps her experiences in the infirmary made her hard and indifferent. But reading the evidence at the hearings and trial it is obvious that among her neighbours at West Auckland there was concern about children and that Mary Ann found it necessary to act concern. And there was her eagerness to observe the proprieties for the dead – the anxiety to have clean linen and white stockings ready for the dead Nattrass; a new nightdress for the baby about to die; a special fruit loaf for the neighbours when the laying-out of little Frederick was over. All this could have been part of her act – needful salving actions – or a simple desire to conform to respectable ritual by the overt side of her duality.

She was never examined to test her sanity – probably this would have been superflous at the time. It was rare for a poisoner to be found insane, especially one such as Mary Ann seems to have been, where there was premeditation, planning, subterfuge – in fact where a clear head was needed, where a course had to be pursued, determination maintained, where any insurrection of pity during a gradual killing had to be smothered, any nervousness controlled or disguised as anxiety for the victim.

The insistence on being the only one in attendance is understandable; the prophetic public expressing of a belief that a victim could well die naturally in the immediate future is fairly common by poisoners. It seems probable that the insurance death-benefits had a part in her calculations. In articles about her, these payments are usually put forward as her reason for poisoning. James Robinson refused to allow her to insure him and he was the only one of her husbands to escape death when with her. And the tampering with building society and post office savings books, and the pledging of articles while she lived with Robinson, is proof of her need or desire for extra money. Gain, at times paltry, is a common reason for poisoning.

Sex is the other common reason. Robinson in any case could have escaped death because Mary Ann seems to have liked living with him. It was Robinson whom she wanted to visit her in prison, not her last lover, Quick-Manning. It was Robinson she mentioned in her prayers. And it was Robinson she turned against bitterly, blaming him for her position. Desire for Joseph

Nattrass, one can assume, was the main reason for Frederick Cotton's death. The chance of living with Cotton was the reason for his sister's death. It is possible that desire for Nattrass contributed to William Mowbray's death. She could have met Nattrass when Mowbray was away at sea, and gone to Seaham when she was free only to find him engaged. Then Nattrass was eventually dispensed with to make way for Quick-Manning, as were, quite possibly, three children. Perhaps the insurance money and opportunity to be with a new lover, or to have some privacy with a husband-lover, operated singly, occasionally jointly. If she did kill to clear the way for marriage to Quick-Manning, which seems pretty certain, it is odd that there was no comment from her about all she had done for him. Perhaps there was, and it was not understood and reported.

But motive for murder very often looks to be inadequate, especially in cases of mass murderers. Helene Jegadi, who poisoned more people than Mary Ann a little before Mary Ann's time, seemed to have genuinely liked some of her victims. Mr Justice Darling, in his charge to the jury in the case of Major Armstrong, executed in 1922, said they would not find a motive which they would regard as adequate, but that did not mean that there was not a sufficient motive for a person with a criminal mind.

That the memorialists protested at the evidence of the other deaths being admitted was understandable, as was the fact that such protest made no impression where it mattered. Even if the evidence had not been admitted, and Mary Ann had been discharged in the Charles Edward trial, the other cases would have followed, and surely, especially on the Nattrass charge, she would not have been cleared of each of them. One she could well have been discharged from would have been that of the baby in whom such a tiny amount of arsenic was found – less than a thousandth of that found in Nattrass. Children, of course, are much more susceptible to the poison. It would seem that Nattrass after a succession of small doses had built up a tolerance to arsenic. The principal effects of arsenic are degeneration of the digestive lining and of other tissues, and often an attack on nerve tissue. This seems to have happened to Nattrass at the end. Among the symptoms are nausea, vomiting, diarrhoea, headaches and muscular pains. Mary Ann seemed to be quite aware that food in the stomach delayed the action of the poison. When the stomach is empty, the effect can be rapid.

The short time the jury was out is also revealing. They were back inside the hour, giving themselves time only to go over the points: there could not have been strong dissension, in spite of the general reluctance to bring in a verdict of guilty against a woman. Also the three days of the trial would give them time to adjust their thinking, away from prior opinion.

But accepting this and respecting much of Campbell Foster's quickly arranged work, her professional defence was far from what it could have been. There was no witness for her at all the preliminary hearings and the trial. The bad start with the despicable George Smith meant she had little chance, especially with the trial so soon after the last magistrates' hearing. Perhaps this is the reason why the case is relatively unknown nationally. Poisonings far less sensational have been written about again and again. If witnesses had been assembled for the defence: if someone had been sought to stand up to Scattergood, her execution would have been far from certain. The *Lancet* did not agree with Scattergood when he said that floating arsenic particles could not get into a person's stomach. Many of the points brought forward in the petitions of Caws, the Sunderland architect, and Nixon, the Darlington solicitor, could have been bases of a powerful defence. No one was thinking for her when it mattered.

One can speculate that she began administering arsenic when she regarded it as a medicine and that a death, accepted by the world as natural, was, she realised, the result of arsenic. Although, if this had been so, one would have expected her to come forward with it as an explanation; but then she said next to nothing, (the law did not then invite a prisoner to give evidence). The beginning, too, how it all started, could have been forgotten: lost in later guilt which she was able to partition off in her mind. There was nothing unusual in regarding arsenic as a medicine. Some people took it as a pick-me-up. Both James Maybrick, the victim in the Maybrick case, and the ill-fated lover L'Angelier in the Madeleine Smith case, were believed to be arsenic eaters. Madeleine Smith used it as a cosmetic.

The Arsenic Act of 1851 stated that arsenic had not to be sold to anyone under twenty-one and the purchaser had to be known to the seller, unless there was a witness known to both. The reason for wanting the arsenic had to be given and the details entered in a special book. In addition, the white powder had to be coloured deliberately; this was done usually with soot or indigo. The practice of selling arsenic mixed with soft soap was common in many areas, as the mixture was used for sheep-dipping. It was possible to soak arsenic from flypapers for many years after the 1851 Act. In the Maybrick case in 1889 more than two grains were obtained from one paper. Arsenical fly-papers also came into the Seddon case in 1912: one of the papers analysed had six grains of arsenic in it. In the Harold Greenwood case in 1920 Marshall Hall had it confirmed by a manufacturing chemist that a seven-pound tin of weedkiller had enough arsenic in it to kill the entire population of Carmarthen. Later Acts have meant that the sale is now closely regulated.

Shocked by Mary Ann's death-throes, a *Newcastle Daily Chronicle* journalist asked how stood the account supposing she was innocent of all but the death of Charles Edward Cotton? He said no one could witness those fierce contortions without a pang of the heart and a wrenching of the nerves. Here was the law of retaliation; the vengeance of the penal code; Christian England demanding an eye for an eye. 'Ache for ache,' he wrote, 'gripe for gripe, pang for pang, torture for torture, she was not released till she had paid the uttermost farthing to the inexorable spirit of public vengeance. Her agonies cried quits, full quits.'

No one could prepare her to face that terrible asphyxiation in the power of the callous and incompetent Calcraft. Her victims suffered, too, although it is highly doubtful if any one of them knew that immediate death was certain and could not be circumvented. But they could have felt innermost dread, and they were denied benefit of clergy, although poor young Frederick Cotton asked for a kindly man to pray with him. The Wesleyan ministers prepared Mary Ann for death, a passing to another life. They were impressed by her, so much so that they were rebuked by the *Durham County Advertiser*, especially Mr Stevenson, who, at her killing, said, 'she is now a saint in Heaven, if ever a woman was.'

West Auckland is still to this day a pleasant place to look at, made so by its fine green – once a popular cricketing venue – and its old-fashioned, stone-built houses. One turns into it from both east and west: travelling west it is the beginning of splendid country, travelling east one knows that the heavily populated part of the county begins round the corner. Just before one reaches that corner there is the workmen's club on the left. It was on this site that Dr Kilburn, unsettled and unhappy as we know for one short period of his life, had his home and surgery. His garden at the back, where the emptied stomach of Charles Edward was temporarily buried, is now built over.

Thomas Riley had his shop at a corner on the other side of the green, the corner of Front Street and Chapel Street; a shop is there still. In his day a pub opposite was splendidly named, Jack in his Glory. He ran a general shop, mainly groceries and clothing, but he also sold medicines; 'druggist' was one of his descriptions. Perhaps his knowledge of powders contributed to his feeling of certainty about Mary Ann. On the same side, right along the green and near its west end, there is a shop, (scheduled for demolition) which once belonged to John Walton Townend, the chemist, where little Charles Edward would see colourful carboys through the small square window panes when he went on his errand for soft soap and arsenic. Townend was also a farmer and kept a large number of horses for hire. His farming could well have caused him to stock a deal of arsenic.

Across the green, standing back quietly on the north side, there is Mary Ann's last home, still well-kept and lived-in. It was here that she stood in the light green doorway early that Friday morning and told Tommy Riley that little Charlie was dead. From her house she would be able to see the corner-shop of her persecutor, with ready-made clothing hanging and swaying outside and in front of it the brewery's excise officer, Quick-Manning, would pass on his way to and from work. Next door was once the Rose and Crown where the inquest was held. Mary Ann's house was used at one time as a dormitory for the pub; a half-door communication was made between the top floors. This is now boarded up. Years before she lived there the ground floor was a barber's shop, 'Barber Bob's'.

The old family house of the Eden family, the Manor House is only a short distance away. The brewery, closed in 1959, is behind this, between it and the modest, quiet Gaunless stream. Beyond, on rising ground, an enormous waste-heap sprawls heavily, grey, smooth-looking, flat-topped, immense, incongruous to behold. This is from the washeries of West Auckland Colliery where Frederick Cotton, Joseph Nattrass and most of the men of Johnson Terrace worked.

Brookfield Cottage, where Quick-Manning was one of Mrs Neasham's gentleman lodgers, is still there, without its name, in Darlington Road, the name now of the orginal Johnson Terrace. Mrs Neasham sent home her servant, Maggie Bell, during Quick-Manning's illness, and later gave her a lustre jug used by Mary Ann to carry milk for Quick-Manning from her own house a few doors away. Maggie Bell's daughter in West Auckland still has the jug.

Another memento, kept by a family in Houghton-le-Spring, is Sergeant Hutchinson's police gloves. Hutchinson achieved some fame because of his part in the case, and his photograph was, at times, attendant to that of Mary Ann. I have not come across illustrations of anyone else in the case. He was awarded a police badge of merit which carried extra pay.

Many of the old houses in Darlington Road, including the one in which Mary Ann lived, are due to be knocked down, but it is obvious that the street, perhaps because of its bright southern aspect, has been a fine one in its day. From the front Mary Ann would see green pastures stretching south, and from the back, looking north, rolling country and gently rounded hills. Scarcely anyone at all realizes that Mary Ann lived there, although that is where four of the five West Auckland deaths took place: even the oldest residents look to the Front Street house, where, in fact, she lived for little over two months. I can think of two reasons for this. The Front Street house was where she was apprehended; it was the house photographed and drawn at the time and subsequent photographers followed suit: it is the house featured on local viewcards down the years, usually with Mary Ann inset wearing a checked shawl and a swathed black bonnet set back on her head and tied with a big taffeta bow. Her smooth, shiny dark hair in front is parted in the centre. The other reason would be uncertainty about Johnson Terrace itself. Not only was it re-named Darlington Road but also its name was switched to Cross Street which ran at an angle to it at the back. The original Johnson Terrace name can (or could) be seen chiselled in a square brown namestone high on the first house of Darlington Road.

The number of Mary Ann's house in Johnson Terrace is not given in the reports or in any documents I have seen. One of the replies I received to a letter in the *Northern Echo* was from a Ferryhill lady who had lived at 20 Darlington Road and who knew that Mary Ann Cotton had lived there before the name switch. I went through the old house as the last resident was bringing out the last of his furniture. Of rough sandstone, it and number nineteen were separated only by an internal centre wall both dowstairs and upstairs. Mary Ann's side faced south. Number nineteen was at the back, and the backyard was shared: it had separate coalhouses and earth closets with brick footrests. There was a passageway, with a kitchen part at the top, from the biggish single downstairs room to the backyard. The window into Darlington Road had a deep sill, as had the windows in the two bedrooms upstairs. These were reached by steepish stairs. The main bedroom was roughly five-by four but the other bedroom, used by Nattrass and William Taylor at one time, was small indeed, only some eight feet square. Of course Nattrass's shift-work meant that often the two men were not using the room at the same time, and I would expect that when William's brother George came to lodge the brothers would share the room and Nattrass would be in the big bedroom with Mary Ann and the children. Why was that seemingly long-desired sleeping together a failure? Because she now had thoughts of making a better marriage with Quick-Manning? That is most probable; and perhaps intimate living with Nattrass was disappointing. Who's to know?

Dr Richardson, who lived in Lanchester Terrace in the village, is remembered wearing his silk hat and frock coat, even in the mornings. The respected Dr Kilburn is remembered in a more endurable way – the splendid west windows of the medieval church of St Helen's Auckland, their deep colours often brilliantly illumined by the afternoon sun, are dedicated to him. The doctor died at the age of fifty-four in 1886, and the windows, triple lancet, within an arch themselves, were erected 'by the parishioners and a few friends,' and inscribed: 'Go and do thou likewise,' and 'Well done thou good and faithful servant.' The ancient church, squat, with a small belfry, is a good half mile from West Auckland, alongside the Bishop Auckland road. Many of the Edens are buried there and somewhere in the graveyard there must be the undiscovered remains of unfortunate Frederick Cotton, as well as the discovered remains of Joe Nattrass, little Charlie and Frederick and of the baby. Nearby the doctor carried out the gruesome dissection.

Mary Ann left two children. I do not know what happened to the elder, the second of her children by Robinson – the baby which was returned to him on New Year's Eve, 1869. New Year's Eve, in the north-east, is a special day: a time of family and personal relationships, when the expressing of them, too embarrassing normally, can be tried and accepted. Families and friends can sometimes achieve a satisfying appreciation of mutual background and experience. And this restless, at times uncomfortable day, when emotions are nearer the surface, intensifies as twelve o'clock approaches. To find his child brought back to him when he returned from watch-night service could have been the most memorable moment of James Robinson's life. Within three years it would be known that the mother was the country's most notorious murderer. How did the child fare in the constant sight of the sorely disappointed and shaken Robinson, and of his sisters who had been suspicious of Mary Ann from the start? One imagines curiosity would not be encouraged.

There was no chance of obscurity for the child born in Durham gaol. Everyone knew that that baby had been taken by a couple of the name of Edwards in Johnson Terrace, West Auckland; and the local people would also know who the father was. There is no indication that he did anything at all for the child. Perhaps he got a job elsewhere – that would be the best way out of it for him. Rumour has it that the child was born blind or became blind; was a fine person; and was paid a halfpenny a day throughout a long life as recompense for being born in prison. There is some truth in this.

In fact the Edwards moved away from West Auckland fairly soon to Leasingthorne, a hamlet some seven miles away, between Bishop Auckland and Ferryhill. Mary Ann's daughter's youngest son told me that he cannot remember his mother talking of living at West Auckland. He referred to Mrs Edwards as Grandma Edwards. Miss Edwards went to school at Leasingthorne and she married early. Her husband was a pitman and there is belief – which could be unfair to him – that he never allowed her to forget her mother's deeds. With their first-born, a daughter, the young couple emigrated to the United States, to a colliery area near to Boston where the husband became a checkweighman. Life in general seems to have been rougher and tougher than in County Durham. A son was born there; then shortly after that, when Mary Ann's daughter was pregnant again, her husband was knocked down and killed by a wagon as he was crossing some lines. She decided to come home to the Edwards. They were then running a pub, the Garden House Hotel, in Low Spennymoor, and her second son was born there. The Edwards made a further move, to the Greyhound Inn in Ferryhill, and there Mary Ann's daughter married again: again to a miner, a hewer at the Dean and Chapter Colliery.

From this marriage a third son was born in Ferryhill in 1901. But she was now plagued with eye trouble, with cataracts, and when she was about thirty she became completely blind. In 1915 her two grown-up sons volunteered for the Army. The younger was killed in June, 1917, at the age of twenty-two, when with the Green Howards. The elder was killed a week before the Armistice, on 4th November, 1918, aged twenty-five, when with the London Rifle Brigade, after being a blighty casualty with the Durhams. When Mary Ann's daughter died in the mid-1950s she was well over eighty, and had been blind for more than fifty years.

Her third son is a good-looking, spruce man who keeps a planned garden immaculately. The distinctive feature in his friendly appearance is his eyes: dark brown, they are bright; they shine. He speaks well of his mother, calling her 'an angel.' She could get about the house on her own, but was usually accompanied outside. So, although it can be thought that fate – with violent deaths for three of her young men and blindness for herself, in addition to her knowledge and others knowing – took some revenge on her because of her mother, she triumphed and came through well. Perhaps she, who began by giving Mary Ann extra life, was, in the end, more like 'a saint in heaven'.

The son she left like his father, was a miner throughout his working life. He retired in 1965 when the Dean and Chapter Colliery at Ferryhill was closed-down. The inland pits are finished or finishing, and his sons are in other work. The Mary Ann Cotton family spanned the lifetime of the Durham coal-field, from pit-sinking to pit closures. The underworld of coal was explored and known far better than the underworld mind of Mary Ann Cotton.

Sources and Acknowledgements

Census Returns (Public and Durham County Record Offices)

Church and civil registers

Home Office file (Public Record Office, London)

Letters in response to mine in the *Northern Echo* and *Sunderland Echo* and following a broadcast

Newpapers of the time: *Durham Chronicle, Durham County Advertiser, Newcastle Courant, Newcastle Daily Chronicle, Newcastle Daily Journal, Northern Echo, Shields Daily News, Sunderland Herald, Sunderland Times, The Times*

Ordnance Survey maps of the time

People spoken to in the West Auckland, East Rainton, South Hetton, Murton and Walbottle areas

Short chapters on Mary Ann Cotton appear in

Richard S. Lambert, *When Justice Faltered* (Methuen, 1935)
Bernard O' Donnell, *Should Women Hang?* (W. H. Allen, 1956)
Patrick Wilson, *Murderess* (Michael Joseph, 1971)

There are factual mistakes in all of these, but this does not invalidate much of the comment

The longest account previous to this book is the earliest, a 91-

page paperback pull-together by an unnamed journalist in 1883 printed by W. J. Cummins, of Market Place, Bishop Auckland. Called *The Life and Career of Mrs Cotton, the West Auckland Poisoner,* it sold at sixpence. It is amazing that this responsible and admirable compilation did not at some time stimulate further research and probing. I have come across only one copy, and that was mutilated with more than a third of its pages missing. I did not see it until this book was with the publishers but I was able to add information which was new to me

Articles on Mary Ann Cotton appear every year or so in north-east newspapers and some of these are filed in local libraries. It was a newspaper article which gave me the idea of writing this book

My copy of Thornton Hall's fanciful tale is five instalments in the weekly *Durham County News* beginning 19th March, 1931. There must be other accounts, probably in women's magazines of many years ago. Writing to me after I had written a radio feature on Mary Ann an eighty-seven-year-old lady in Bradford said my story was not quite correct and that the truth which she had read was that Mary Ann took in unwanted babies for a fee and then killed them by drawing the breath from their bodies

There is also the melodrama, *Mary Ann Cotton.* With its comedy spots this was played in the north-east as late as between the wars.

Books I have referred to include:

Criminal Law Cases, Vol. XII, Northern Circuit, Reg. v Cotton
Dictionary of National Biography
John Glaister, *The Power of Poison* (Chris. Johnson, 1954)
J. D. J. Havard, 'The Detection of Secret Homicide', *Cambridge Studies in Criminology,* Vol. VI (Macmillan, 1960)
W. Arthur Moyes, *Mostly Mining* (Frank Graham, 1969)
John Deane Potter, *The Fatal Gallows Tree* (Elek, 1965)
William Robinson, *The Story of the Royal Infirmary, Sunderland* (Hills, 1934)
Sidney James Webb, *The Story of the Durham Miners* (Fabian Society, 1921)
Directories of the time; local guide books and county books

The bulk of the paper research was done in the Durham County Record Office and in the Sunderland and Newcastle Central Libraries Reference rooms. I am most grateful for their store of information and for the repeated help from their patient staffs. I spent a few days in the Public Record Office in London and some time at Somerset House; in Registrar's offices in the north-east and in the Northumberland County Record Office. In addition to the church registers I worked through in the Durham Record Office I was given access to the registers of St Andrew's church, Dalton-le-Dale; St Andrew's church, Newcastle and St Mary's church, West Rainton.

The letters I received after mine appeared in the *Northern Echo* and *Sunderland Echo* led me to Mary Ann's grandson; to her first house in West Auckland; and to knowledge of her address in Pallion when she was married to Robinson. A broadcast following one of the published letters brought me further information including the loan of letters written to Mary Ann in Durham gaol.

Many people have been kind enough to help me and I am grateful. They include Mr and Mrs Alderson of West Auckland, Mr Arthur Almond of Durham, Mrs Bailes of West Auckland, Mr J. G. Crowder of South Hetton who sent me the version of the children's rhyme I have used, Mr George Hall of Murton, Mrs Romola D. Hicks of Chardstock, Devon, Mrs M. A. Lundy of Shildon, Mrs M. J. Marshall of Chilton, Mr Sidney Monk of West Auckland, the Revd E. B. Pateman of Murton, Mr Dixie Pritchard of West Cornforth, Mrs K. Riddell of Sunderland, the Revd W. J. Taylor of Sunderland, Mr G. D. Thompson of Redcar, Mr John Wackett of Darlington who generously sent me photocopies of his own newspaper research, Miss Jennie Wade of Annfield Plain, Mr James A. Weatherley of Walbottle, the Revd E. Welsh of West Rainton and Mr G. Wyvill of Sunderland.

Finally my thanks to Mary Ann's grandson who could have sent me packing but didn't.

Index

Appleton, Mr (warder), 133
Archibald, Sir Thomas Dickson *(Judge)*, 68, 70, 71, 73, 78, 79, 80, 82, 84, 85, 87-90, 93-100, 102, 110, 116; summing-up 97-99
Armstrong, Lt Col. Charles *(prison governor)*, 69, 70, 101, 104, 108, 116, 117, 130, 139
Armstrong, Major, case, 139
Arsenic, 19, 20, 23, 24, 27, 34, 35, 39, 40, 42-6, 53, 57, 66, 73, 78-81, 83, 86-96, 98, 104, 112, 113, 115, 116, 136, 139, 140-1, 142
Aspinall, Mr, *(QC)*, 68, 70, 71
Atkinson, Elijah *(witness)*, 34, 38, 39
Atkinson, Elizabeth *(witness)*, 36, 39
Avory, Mr Justice, 136

Backhouse, Edward, 63, 64, 111, 114, 115, 117
Barnard Castle, 111
Bax, Canon Arthur Nesham, 58
Bede, The Venerable, 56
Bell, Maggie, 142-3
Bennett, Revd J, 126-7, 130
Bethune, Revd, 108
Bishop Auckland, 12, 19, 21-4, 27, 28, 29, 31-45, 46, 71, 76, 85, 110, 118, 130
Bishop of Dover, 127
Blackwell, Mr, 30, 69, 110
Booth, Mary Ann, *(arsenic-purchaser)*, 40
Bousfield, William, 122
Bowser, Richard *(Under Sheriff)*, 71, 101, 130, 131, 133
Boyd,William *(prison surgeon)*, 27, 132, 133
Broadbent, Dr Samuel, 52
Bruce, Gainford *(assisting prosecution counsel)*, 68, 74
Bruce, Henry Austin, later *Lord Aberdare (Home Secretary)*, 24, 26, 27, 29-30, 64, 101,108, 111, 113-7, 132
Burns, Mr *(Robinson's brother-in-law)*, 110-11

Calcraft, William, 121-2, 125-6, 128-32, 134, 136, 141
Carmarthen, 141
Carr, Mrs, 82
Caws, Frank *(petitioner)*, 115-6, 140
Chalmers, Dr Archibald, 15, 16, 18, 20, 23, 39, 41, 42, 44, 74, 77, 81-2, 88, 96, 99, 112
Chapman, Charles, 27-8, 30, 37
Clayton, Canon, 65
Coleridge, Sir John Duke *(Attorney-General)*, 68, 71
Common, A. W. *(J. P.)* 114
Cornwall, 51, 54
Cotton, Mrs Adelaide, 65
Cotton, Charles *(London)*, 65, 67, 77
Cotton,Charles Edward *(boy)*, 14-15; inquest 16-19, 20; first hearing of case 21-4, 28, 33, 43-5, 65; trial 68-101; 106, 111, 120, 125, 139, 141, 142, 144
Cotton, Frederick *(husband, bigamous)*, 13, 14, 16, 25-6, 32, 51, 62-7, 72, 91, 93, 94, 106-7, 135, 139, 142, 144
Cotton, Frederick *(boy)*, 14; committal hearing 37-41; 42, 43, 44, 72, 74, 86, 88, 91, 138, 141, 144
Cotton, Margaret, 44, 64-6, 135
Cotton, Margaret Edith Quick-Manning *(baby, prison-born)*, 11-12, 29, 117-20, 122-3, 127, *(grown-up)* 145-6
Cotton, Mary Ann, *(also Robson, Mowbray, Ward and Robinson)*, prologue 11-12; murders at West Auckland 13-20, first hearing of Charles Edward Cotton's murder 21-4; other committal hearings 29-46; early life 47-50; as Mrs Mowbray 50-4; as Mrs Ward 55-8; meets and marries Robinson 58-64; and Cotton 64-7; Assizes 68-101; letters from prison

29, 102-3, 105-7, 109, 110, 123; the hanging 125-34; summary 135-46; her grandson 145-6, 149
Cotton, Robert Robson*(baby)*, 14, 27, 32; committal hearing 41-3; 44, 45, 50, 66, 67, 72, 86, 87, 88, 91, 95, 139, 144
Cowl, Mr *(doctor's assistant)*, 56
Crooks, Mr, 130

Daily News, The, 104
Darling, Mr Justice, 139
Darlington, 111, 115, 134
Davison, William *(witness)*, 77
Dean, Thomas, *(deputy coroner)*, 16, 73
Detchon, Thomas, *(chemist's assistant)*, 40, 43, 44, 72
Dixon, Dr, 56-7
Dodds, Mary Ann *(witness)*, 18, 19, 21-2, 28-9, 73-5, 94
Dolan, John, 133
Douglas, Mary, 29
Drummond, Joseph, 26
Dun Well pit, East Rainton, 49
Durham, 11, 24, 26, 27, 31, 45, 46, 68-101, 117, 121, 125, 127, 129, 134
Durham Chronicle, 26
Durham County Advertiser, 24, 28, 103-4, 125, 132, 135, 137, 141
Durham Gaol, 21, 24, 27-9, 31, 36, 40, 43, 45, 69, 71, 101-34. 145
Durham General Sessions, 46

Easby, Dr, 24
East Rainton, 47-9
Eden family, The, 142, 144
Edwards, Miss, 145-6
Edwards, Sarah and William, 118-20, 122, 123, 127, 145
Elliott, Mr J F., 103
Evens, Robert *(assistant hangman)*, 126, 128, 130, 131, 134
Everest, George *(Home Office)*, 132
Exhumations, 19-20, 24-6, 39, 42, 88

Favell, John *(coroner)*, 133
Fawcett, Mr, 103, 119
Ferryhill, 145-6
Foster, Thomas Campbell *(defending counsel)*, 46, 71-89; closing address 94-6, 98, 99, 110, 140
Friendly Societies Select Committee Report of 1854, 85

Gallon, Frances and Joseph, 66
Gammage, Dr, 53, 54
Garner case, 85
Geering, Mary Ann, case, 85, 86, 89, 116
Gladstone, Mr W. E., 68, 70, 114
Green, Robert *(petitioner)*, 115
Greener, T. *(jury foreman)*, 99
Greenhow, Mr *(assistant to Russell)*, 68, 74, 75, 86, 110
Greenwood, Harold, case, 141

Hale, H., 108
Hall, Colonel, 31, 35-7, 43
Hall, Sir Edward Marshall, 141
Hall, George, 107-8
Hall, Matthew, 124
Hall, Thomas *(witness)*, 32
Hall, Thornton, 53, 63, 148
Hardy, Dr, 96-7
Hays, John, 121, 126, 128-9, 133
Hazard pit, East Rainton, 47, 48, 49
Hedley, George *(witness)*, 33, 34, 36, 68
Hedley, Jane *(witness)*, 33, 36, 38, 40-1, 44, 88
Heffernan, Dr, 66
Henderson, Superintendent John, 19, 20, 2, 36, 60
Henderson, Mrs, 36
Hetton Lyons pit, 49
Hick, Revd W. James, 21, 23, 31
Hodgson, Major, 31, 36, 40
Holdforth, Henry, 105-7, 109, 124
Holt case, 85
Holy Trinity Church, South Hetton, 52, 53
Home Office, The, 19, 25, 26, 27, 30, 60, 102, 113, 116-7, 132, 133
Howard Association, The, 132
Huddleston, Mr T.C., 108
Hulbard, Mr and Mrs John *(uncle and aunt)*, 53, 110
Humphrey, Mr, 57, 58
Hutchinson, Sergeant Tom, 15-6, 19, 207 26, 29, 35, 39, 65, 67, 88, 112, 143

Insurance, 15, 24, 25, 32, 34, 40-1, 44, 54, 59, 61, 67, 72, 85-6, 93, 104, 138, 139; burial clubs 137

Jegadi, Helene, 139
Jellis, Miss *(wardress)*, 130
Jobson, Mr J, 21, 31

Kilburn, Dr, 15-16, 18-20, 22-5, 35, 38, 39,

41, 42, 44, 72, 73, 76-83, 88, 91, 99, 112, 120, 141, 144

Labron, Thomas, 69-70, 102, 105
Lancet, The, 112-3, 140
L'Angelier, M., 140
Lankester, Dr *(Camden Town coroner)*, 137
Leng, John, 46
Liddell, Hon A. F. O. *(Home Office)*, 102, 116-7
Life and Death of Mary Ann Cotton (play), 134
Low Moorsley, 47, 48
Lowe, Revd J.C. *(prison chaplain)*, 111, 120, 126, 130, 133
Lowlands, George 133
Lowrey, William *(lodger)*, 17, 18, 28, 29, 68, 119, 122-3, 133

McConville, John, 133
McKieve, Mrs, 86
Maling, Dr Edward Allan, 56, 57, 63, 111, 114
Marshall, Mr E.G., 130
Marshall, Mr H. I., 26
Marwood, William, 121
Maughan, Mr and Mrs, 122
Maybrick case, 140, 141
Moore, George, 102-3, 105
Moore, Joseph, 133
Mountford, Revd J. M., 126, 127, 130
Mowbray, Isabella *(daughter)*, 25, 52, 54, 59-60, 61, 63, 107, 135
Mowbray, John Robert *(son)*, 53
Mowbray, Margaret Jane *(daughter)*, 52
Mowbray, Margaret Jane 11 *(daughter)*, 52, 54, 55
Mowbray, Mary Ann *(daughter)*, 52
Mowbray, William *(husband)*, 25, 50-4, 94, 106, 108, 135, 138, 139
Murray, Charles, 37, 68-9
Murton Colliery, 25, 48-52, 105, 108

Napier, Sir William, 114
Nattrass, Joseph *(lover)*, 13-4, 16, 24, 28; committal hearing 32-6, 41, 42, 43, 45, 54, 69, 76, 86-7, 89, 90, 91, 95, 112, 135, 137, 138-9, 142, 144
Neasham, Mrs, 142
Newcastle-upon-Tyne, 13, 32, 40, 44, 51, 66, 77, 137
Newcastle Daily Chronicle, 99, 116, 126, 132, 135, 141
Newcastle Journal, 17, 19, 103-5, 108, 135
Newcastle Register Office, 51
Newgate, 121, 122, 125
Nicholson, Mary, 46, 129
Nixon, John T. *(petitioner)*, 111-3, 140
North Walbottle, 13, 44, 65-7
Northern Echo, 104, 111, 119-20, 123, 132, 136, 143, 149
Norwich, 121

Olive, Martha *(petitioner)*, 113-4
O'Reilly, Bernard, 112
O'Reilly, L. Delmar, 112
Owen, William, 40

Pallion, Sunderland, 25, 40, 58-63, 109
Parr, William, 76
Part, Mr *(assistant to Foster)*, 71
Peace, Charles, 71
Pease and Partners, 16
Penzance, 51, 52
Petitions, 111-7, 122, 132, 139
Police report, 25-6, 48, 60
Pollock, Baron, 85
Post-mortem examinations, 16, 18-9, 22-3, 24, 27
Potter, Edward and Margaret, 50, 54, 64, 137
Priestley, Mary *(witness)*, 77
Quick-Manning, Mr *(lover)*, 13-4, 15, 16, 17-8, 22, 28, 38, 75,76, 77, 86, 87, 138, 139, 142, 144

Ranson, Alderman George Smith *(petitioner)*, 114-5
Reinsch's test, 19, 73, 78
Richardson, Dr Thomas Charlton, 32-5, 87, 112, 137, 144
Riley, Thomas *(accuser)*, 14-17, 22-5, 35, 44, 75, 93, 104, 105, 120, 142
Robinson, Elizabeth *(child)*, 59-60,
Robinson, Mrs Hannah, 58
Robinson, James *(husband)*, 13, 25, 26, 40, 44, 58-62, 64, 66, 106-11, 125, 127, 135, 138, 144-5
Robinson's sisters, 60, 106-7, 145
Robinson, James *(child)*, 59-60
Robinson, John *(baby)*, 58-9, 63
Robinson, Margaret *(prison matron)*, 31, 123, 130
Robinson, Mary Isabella *(daughter, baby)*,60
Robinson, Miss *(wardress)*, 130
Robson, Elizabeth *(Newcastle)*, 40, 44

Robson, Margaret *(mother, later Mrs George Stott)*, 47-8, 50, 51, 52, 54, 59, 124, 126, 135
Robson, Margaret *(sister)*, 47-8
Robson, Michael *(father)*, 25, 47-51, 106, 126
Robson, Phoebe *(witness)*, 32, 38, 42, 86,
Robson, Robert *(brother)*, 14, 48, 50, 106
Robson, W. W., 116
Russell, Charles, *(Q.C.)*, 45, 68, 70, 71, 72, 73-7, 80, 82-5, 88-9; closing address 90-4, 95, 100, 110, 115

St Andrew's Church, Dalton-le-Dale, 52
St Andrew's Church, Newcastle, 13, 51, 66
St Helen's Auckland Church, 18, 20, 24, 25-6, 144
St Oswald's Church, Durham, 127, 129
St Mary's Church, West Rainton, 477 48
St Peter's Church, Sunderland, 55-6
Sans Street Mission Hall, Sunderland, 58, 63
Scattergood, Dr Thomas, 20, 23, 24, 35, 39-40, 42, 73, 78, 83-5, 88, 89, 91-92, 96, 98, 112-3, 140
Seaham, 54, 108, 125, 139
Seddon, Frederick, case, 141
Shafto, Revd A. D., 120
Shaw, Dr, 59-60
Shaw family, 13
Slane, Hugh, 121, 126, 128-9, 133
Smith, George F, 27-30, 36-7, 68-9, 105-6, 110, 123, 130, 140
Smith, Isabella *(witness)*, 74
Smith, Madeleine, case, 140
Smith, Sarah *(witness)*, 33, 38, 39, 41-2, 45, 74, 76, 94
Smith, Thompson *(head warder)*, 31, 36-7, 130
Smyrna House, *Home for Fallen Women*, 64, 111
Society of Friends, 115, 122
South Hetton, 25, 49, 50-4, 62, 108, 111, 124
Spennymoor, 44, 63, 66-7, 121, 145
Stevenson, Revd W., 120-3, 127, 130, 141
Stott, George *(stepfather)*, 50, 107, 125, 127
Stott, John, 108
Stott, Margaret *(wife of John)*, 108, 111, 133-4, *her grand-daughter* 108
Stubbs, Jane, 108
Sunderland, 25, 40, 46, 53-64, 67, 74, 109-10, 111, 114-6, 138; Infirmary 54-6, 61, 74; School of Art and Design, 63
Sunderland Times, 26, 114, 116, 135
Surtees, Colonel *(High Sheriff)*, 71

Tallack, William *(Home Office)*, 114-15, 132
Tate, Mary *(witness)*, 33, 41, 42, 44, 45, 76-7, 86
Taylor, George *(lodger)*, 14, 72, 86, 87, 94, 144
Taylor, William *(lodger)*, 14, 72, 86, 94, 144
Taylor on Evidence, 85
Thubron, Mary *(Mrs Nattrass)*, 54
Times, The, 70-1, 90, 132
Townend, John Walton *(chemist)*, 22, 73, 75, 96, 142
Trewhitt's Building Society, 61
Trotter, William Dale *(Clerk to the Justices)*, 19, 24, 25, 26-7, 29-30, 31, 32, 35-7

Vacquier, Jean Pierre *(trial of)*, 136
Vickers, George *(witness)*, 32

Ward, George *(husband)*, 25, 55-8, 60, 63, 74, 94, 135
Wayman's Building Society, 61
Wesleyan Methodists, 48, 49, 50, 58, 120-8, 137, 144
West Auckland, 12, 13-20, 25, 45, 46, 62, 94, 109,138, 141-3; Colliery 13, 32, 142
West Hartlepool, 134
West Hartlepool Phrenological Society, 133
Wheelhouse, Mr *(M.P.)*, 70

Young, James *(deputy prison governor)*, 130, 133
Young, James *(witness)*, 40-1

Postscript

September, 1996

Of the two of her children (from twelve) who survived Mary Ann I wrote of the one who, growing within her, delayed the trial, entered the world outside in the larger womb of a prison destined to discard her, and duly ten weeks later she was wrenched away leaving her mother to be hanged. This child who became blind in her late twenties, had at least four children, three of them boys, the two eldest killed in the First World War, at the ages of twenty-two and twenty-five. I met this woman's remaining son, a good-looking, retired Durham miner. I did not know at the time whether or not Mary Ann's other child, her second one to James Robinson, had lived. Some years later, when I was tutor at a local authority evening class in Sunderland, one of the students, a male nurse, mentioned that a colleague had said that she was a descendant of Mary Ann Cotton. 'What's her name?' I asked. 'Robinson,' he said. This led me to her father, where I had further luck - we had worked in the same engineering shop at Deptford in Sunderland forty years previously.

James Robinson was Mary Ann's third and last legitimate husband - her real name at the end was Mary Ann Robinson - and he was left with three children, two, a boy and girl, by his previous wife, and I needed to check that my old workmate was not a descendant of this boy. With candour he assured me that he wasn't, that he was the great grandson of Mary Ann, the grandson of the baby, George Robinson, she walked away from, leaving it with a friend who on New Year's Eve 1869 presented it to the father.

His grandfather had done well, becoming a manager at Short Brothers' shipyard at Pallion, adjacent to where James Robinson and Mary Ann had their home; lived for a time in style in Northumberland and left some property in Deptford. Two of his sisters went to Australia. He died about 1921. His son, my friend's father, would not allow any talk of Mary Ann.

George, born 18 June 1869, is entered in the 1871 census aged one, and in the 1881 census, when the Robinsons were still in Rosanna Street, Deptford but in a different house, eleven year old George had a younger sister aged nine. No wife to Robinson is entered. This child would be born about 1872 when Mary Ann was alive, and this proof of another liaison may have been a contributory reason for Robinson's reluctance to visit Mary Ann in prison. She asked him to visit her with the three children (childer), and although he turned up - without the children - he failed to summon up courage to face her, and his companion, his brother-in-law, did so in his stead.

I was brought up in Pallion, in High Pallion, at the top of the bank to the river and the shipyards. In the territory-conscious world of boys, for me to penetrate into the few segregated streets of Low Pallion was risky unless escorted, but I know that I ventured into Grace Street at least once. I heard of Mary Ann when I was a boy, but I was not aware of any deep emotive local memory of her, despite the highly probable four poisonings she did at Pallion. There could well have been such memory retained in the small cut-off community of Low Pallion. I was to find it in mining villages where she lived, captured in children's rhymes and mythical tales - that she ran a baby-farm, that she pushed a boy or young man down a shaft. The latter was repeated so confidently I wondered if it were true. My living in Pallion had nothing to do with my decision to write about her. this followed the shock of rejection of a long-worked-at novel. I read a feature in the press about her, thought the tale sensational, and found that it had not been conscientiously researched. I had been a news reporter and felt that if this story was not worth publishing I must have no idea of what was out of the ordinary. On seeing some early work on it, three publishers were interested, but none commissioned it - it was obvious that I was going to finish the job. Michael Joseph Limited was the most promising. They took the completed script quite quickly.

I was and still am bemused by this lone stealthy killer, the ultimate traitor to those close to her, but when she faced her own killing I was shocked that the hoped for, the expected, instant transition to a better world became three minutes or so of strangulation. I could understand why reporters were later barred from witnessing hangings. Without the hysteria of public hangings - these were ended in 1868 - they could remain level headed and tell how it was. They were representing the public. I don't think Mary Ann's hanging was all that exceptional.

Throughout the centuries a quick hanging has not been the intention. That such was beyond the ability of the hangman was of no consequence. A slow one was part of the punishment. The traitorous high born have been grateful that they were to be beheaded, accepting the risk of blunt blades and nervous executioners. Take these guineas, my executioner, and please, please see that your axe is sharp. Traitors were cut down after some minutes of hanging when they were still alive so that further dire things could be done. In normal hangings it was usual to leave the body hanging for an hour. Even as recently as the judicial hanging of Nazis, Pierrepoint, who prided himself on clean executions, and was pleased when he dispatched eleven before lunch, had two men at the bottom of the drop to pull the legs. Before Pierrepoint's days death from hanging was usually the result of strangulation and asphyxia. In 1864, nine years before William Calcraft bungled Mary Ann's execution, the Commission on Capital Punishment heard that his methods were 'very rough, much the same as if he had been hanging a dog.'

In 1975 the BBC in Newcastle put out, *A Slight Case of Poison*, three half hours based on the book in which the actress who took the part of Mary Ann made the playing of her role difficult as she believed that Mary Ann was innocent. The book provoked John Downie to write a long imaginative play, *Mary Ann: An Elegy* concentrating on events in West Auckland in the two weeks before she was arrested. Howard Davies directed members of the Royal Shakespeare Company in a rehearsed reading of this at the Warehouse in October 1977. Downie cut the play to last inside two hours and it was staged at the 1979 Edinburgh Festival by Bristol Express The full version was published by July Fox of Bristol in 1979. The book is also used ingeniously by Terry Deary in his novel *Shadow Play*, (Scholastic Publications 1992), in which the Mary Ann Cotton story becomes an integral part, part of the core, of the writing.

Recently, in 1996, Tony Whitehead of Seaham produced a documentary record of Mary Ann. He has assembled many vital certificates and he queries some of my conclusions on the number of probable poisonings. He discovered the address in Sunderland to which Mary Ann and her first husband William Mowbray moved from South Hetton. It was Henry Street East in Hendon. Mowbray was going to sea then and could scarcely have chosen a home nearer to it. Their son, John Robert William, was born and died there, and Mowbray died there too, at another house in the same street. The street is still there but the residential houses have gone. It is a reconstructed industrial street, one side all one long factory. the other a miscellany. Should the ghost of Dr Gammage flit along the street now it might quiver at the car radios or portable radios accompanying working motor mechanics in deference to the time when the doctor, it is said, stopped when he heard Mary Ann singing after the death of her husband.

Films and television can't be blamed for putting ideas into Mary Ann's head. She could have become alienated. Her stepfather was no comparable replacement for her real father. There was the shame of a Sunday School teacher becoming pregnant before marriage, the recourse to a register office marriage in distant impersonal big Newcastle, and then the lonely life in the southwest with Mowbray out all day. Maybe that was the time when she felt the world had turned against her and a secret hardness began, a hardness which endured even when she returned to the warmth of colliery life. Where did she pick up her knowledge of arsenic? The southwest? Certainly I think prior to working at the Fever Hospital in Sunderland. Arsenic was used medicinally in small doses; even Chekhov, a doctor as well as a writer, used it. Yet I fancy if its killing power had accidentally appeared she would have told of this. Her silence is against her. She did not protest enough. Surely she was independent enough to throw off the rascally Smith's injunction not to speak, but she did not.

Mary Ann was brought down by Riley, as well she knew: 'As fore Riley god Will judge him, not A orthely Juge.' I have wondered at the persistence of the man who had no support from the doctors in West Auckland, from the police, or from anyone. I have spoken frequently about Mary Ann over the years and in Bishop Auckland I found there were people who had thought about Riley, and were of the opinion that his unrelenting bitter suspicion of Mary Ann had been fuelled because she had rejected his advances ... and he a man who could put work her way. He would regard it as an affront. It is possible.